I0123939

Pranic Self-Healing

INTENTION not In Tension

Llan Starkweather

A journalog or chronicle of ongoing healing in an altered state of conscious awareness transcending the inhibiting parameters of thought and belief

Published by the Wizard at Lulu.com
First Edition   June 2007
Copyright by Llan Starkweather. All rights reserved
ISBN 978-0-6151-5093-2

Author's website   Llanscaping.org
Email   Llan@hughes.net

Previous books:
Edgehouse – Embracing the Energies of Change
The Railroad that Changed Leverett Forever
All-That-Is Waving – In Resonance with the Vibes

PreFacing if this is for you

Pranic Self-Healing is clearly a work in progress. I chronicle as best I can what I experience, as I started doing 30 years ago for my voracious self audience, and this pranic access to the body energy stream becomes for me more and more readily available. These last few months I've given full and rather bizarre demonstrations of tension-free vibrations with simultaneous accompanying explanatory commentary to anybody in my soul family circle willing to set aside their own drama for a while to listen, as a family with an unconditional contract has learned to do. I mention here my 29-year Men's Family group of 10 with whom I have shared more quality time than any entity else, meeting the entire third Sunday of each month for 29 years with periodic 4-day retreats. They are entity-bound with my reportage of my experience in these altered states as our group started with one such rather mild state in 1978 and since never departed from our each viewing life every day with new eyes.

I entered the new age of self discovery in middle age in the 70s and have learned doctrines and have studied and followed channeler's and guru's ideas and therapies from you name it, recording in 1976 a mind shift mentioned below that caused several close biological relatives to set my relation-ship to them adrift. I was actively involved in a 3-year dis-covery Internet group mid-nineties seeking to test and codify the altered state called *ayahuasca*'s ingredients from the 106 herbs used in *ayahuasca* ritual by 160 Central American societies. Along the way, group 'moderator' Terence McKenna brought DMT to my house, created nurseries in Hawaii, learned that we generate DMT, found to be one of the two active components of *ayahuasca*, in our spinal columns 3 to 5 am and are as 'high' as we normally get from it, especially when the other ingredient was found to be an MAO Inhibitor, which we also generate. In the *ayuhasca* herbal, that second significant MAO Inhibiting plant sets aside your body's DMT controls in relationship to serotonin, endorphins and such much more than your own night-time regulation thereof does (it turned out that the mind-control government couldn't control *ayahuasca* as reformulated. Not only were we 'holding' every night *in corpum*, but the best DMT source found, after obtaining, growing, and testing all the designat-ed plants we could scavenge, was a *phalaris* grass that sheep farmers in the Southwest disliked for its affects on their wards, and *Syrian rue*, a seed from Middle Eastern grocery stores and the red dye of Oriental rugs, provides the most powerful MAO Inhibitor). All this information in the form of FAQs and trip reports is stored at the **Lycaeum.org** which we created at the time.

Anybody who's going to get anything out of this book probably needs to have some of my sort of Seeking Credentials and possibly advanced age (or be what my daughter Meg calls 'an old soul') in order to have discovered that **the *witness* and the *will* are pale sisters of *intention*, the energy of realization**.

Somewhere below, I talk about the inner dialog of doubt that surfaces when you realize with *intention* your arrival in a place that you hitherto have not believed in. A discyple to *intention* knows this dialog of doubt and disregards it, blindly moving forward and in altered consciousness even if doubting time's parameters – riding the belch of change that is currently ever more available to rampant open curiosity concerning life's porpoise. What follows includes an examination of where curiosity has led me and report snippets from altered moments of body consciousness to help you to steer your own unique course of self-rediscovery. Nothing really wraps up this section of the book at its end, because discovery isn't finished.

Master Cho in his book has provided the basic opening to these body energies with dozens of exercises for sharpening your focus to the auric flows and is promoting the healing of others. I don't think the *protocol* needs to be that complex once you get a grasp on your *intentions*. His approach is all about identifying and manipulating the energy like massage and manually removing "contamination or dirty energy" from your aura, while my introduction to fully sensing the flowing vibrations of embodyment and to riding them to adjuvenation is a much bigger piece. Identifying and vibrating small or larger energy complexes and moving consciousness into them restores a balance to them that has been lost in adjusting to life's developmental challenges. I don't believe the body's centering self-therapies like tai chi, focusing on controlling the body's opposing forces, can restore the auric natal balance of free energy flow. **The body yearns towards health and replaces almost all of its components on a regular schedule, but the patterning of that ongoing restoration must be returned to its youthful balance, which *intention* can accomplish.**

psi Energy
The Geometry of Consciousness

It is an illusion that there is a space between us and the universe that we live in. There is no separation between mind and body, mind and mind, mind and world - **the essence of our nature is consciousness**. The psychic abilities collectively known as **psi**, from the Greek word for soul, destroy this illusion of separation. **Extrasensory perception**, or ESP, provides one connection to this mystery located between space and time. The ESP companion, "**spiritual healing**, reveals the powerful effects that our consciousness can have in the presence of peaceful receptivity, trust, and loving intentions." David Bohm says "a change in meaning is a change in being" concerning thought's effects on the physical and psychic world. A mystic might call the informational exchange of spiritual healing "universal love".

Twelfth-century Buddhist Dzogchen teachings advise us to look directly at our awareness and experience **the geometry of consciousness - the relationship of our awareness to the space-time in which we live.** These teachings of expanded awareness and the experience of spaciousness are not about self-improvement or gaining power; they are about self-realization: discovering who we really are. In developing psychic abilities which can reveal that the self or ego is not who we actually are - one of them being the practice of **remote viewing** [earlier described as **'prophesy'**] we discover through the process that we ourselves are the flow of loving awareness that is available to us whenever we are quiet and peaceful.

The choices we make as individuals determine which mansion or quantum possibilities we experience in our personal lives. **We may all have latent psi powers, but our ability to develop them is being blanked out by socially engineered stress, with the collusion of covert agencies**.

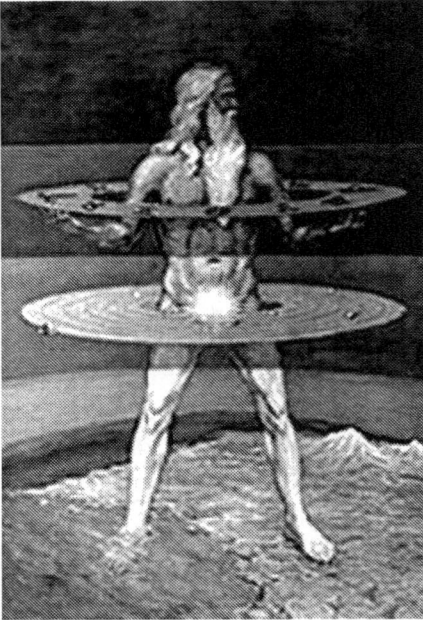

We have the evidence of a powerful technology,

forgotten long ago hidden deep within our collective memories. The events observed in the world around us mirror the development of beliefs within. Rather than **creating our reality**, it may be more accurate to say that we create the conditions into which **we attract future outcomes**, already established, into focus in the present.

We all have it in us to travel back and forth between the two orders of the primary implicate order or quantum hologram of the mind that is Minding and transcends all specification - knowing neither 'here' nor 'there' - and the decoded unfolded reality manifest in our space and time. Think of local consciousness on the electromagnetic spectrum of light as the foreground and the quantum mind as the background. We all have the capacity to enlarge and open the doors of our perception to receive news of the universe. Operating at higher frequencies within the electromagnetic spectrum of the light domain, we become citizens of a larger universe in regard to perception, time, space, dimensionality, and possibility. Our psychological make-up is less trauma-tized by past experience, is more capacious and capricious, and we feel extended into a multi-dimensional universe.

All life begins on the edge, a place of opportunity, of change and spaciousness, information, excitement, and new possibilities. A mystic is on the edge in consciousness. When we find ourselves truly on the edge, there is an opportunity for an event, a spiritual teacher, or a friend - even a book - to pry loose the fingers of limitation and set us free.

Based on meticulous research at the prestigious yet malevolent Stanford Research Institute (SRI) during the early 70s, the almost forgotten science of **prophesy** as a respected profession is clad in a new name, **remote viewing**, a process where you can quiet your mind and **inflow** information from anywhere in the essentially holographic world. Similarly, you can **outflow** your intentions to heal or relieve the pain of a distant person in **distant healing**.

Spatially separate events are shown to be not independent and demonstrate the non-local nature of our universe. Our minds have access to events occurring in distant places - and even into the future. **In 277 formal remote-viewing research trials by SRI and Princeton University it was found no harder to describe tomorrow's remote viewing target location than it is to describe today'**s. Eminent researcher Russell Targ (co-founder of the SRI International remote-viewing ESP program and pioneer in the development of the laser) says that "Data from the past 25 years have shown that a remote viewer can answer any question about events anywhere in the past, present, or future, and be correct more than two-thirds of the time. For an experienced viewer, the rate of correct answers can be much higher."

Though the specifics may vary from person to person, the general procedure is similar for each viewer. A quiet mental place in the present moment, in the now, is found on the edge between the inflow and the outflow - "the peace that passeth understanding". This is an archetypal feeling of non-separation from all of humanity and nature. In this place of limitless mind, one can visit non-local existence beyond space and time. Often beginning in a mild, closed eye state of relaxation, the receiver works with sensory impressions regarding events that may be occurring anywhere on the planet - in the next room or half way around the globe. Trained to distinguish among the many kinds of sensations, the viewer then assigns identifiers to the experience, refining the impressions to greater levels of detail. Sounds, smells, tastes, and sensations as well as images, may accompany such a journey. **The training that teaches remote viewers to accept and record such impressions without bias is the expertise that sets them apart from the casual dreamer**.

Rigid scientific study and serious investigations of the last 50 years have shown that all of spacetime is available to one's consciousness, which is always non-located on the edge of the awareness of an individual. This entirely new realm of secret intelligence gathering with fewer risks (now it is assumed somewhat replaced with satellite surveillance) has 'scientifically' confirmed the principles of such inner technology, understood by prophets 2,500 years ago.

Only recently declassified, SRI remote-viewing experiments provided dramatic proof of the existence and utilization of non-local mind in CIA "espionage" during the Cold War.

Edgar Cayce, the 'sleeping prophet'. offered a key to the science of prophecy, reminding us that we indeed influence the course of history through the course of our lives in the present. Our responses to the challenges of our lives may determine, at least in part, the degree to which we experience the changes he foresaw. "It may depend upon much that deals with the metaphysical... There are those conditions that in the activity of individuals, in line of thought and endeavor, keep oft many a city and many a land through their application of spiritual laws."

Regardless of whose visions or prophesies into the future we consider, for the most part each appears to escape exact measurement of time. They appear to represent moments of possibility, rather than concrete appointments with a precise outcome. Neither ancient nor current prophesies can predict our future; **we are refining our choices every moment!** While we may appear to be on one path destined for a specific outcome, our path can change radically to produce another outcome that is quite unexpected. Gregg Braden, in the Isaiah Effect, says that "Quantum physics suggests that the opportunity to redefine outcomes may come only at specific intervals where the roads of time *bend their courses* and approach other roads. Sometimes the roads move so close that they touch one another" These points of touch between parallel universes are "windows of opportunity choice points". Physicists now believe that matter is made of many short bursts, rather than being one continuous field.

The ancients believed that time occurred in a similar fashion. **Seth said we were blinking on and off**. It is during these bursts of light quanta that create our reality that we experience the events of our world. The more bursts of light we string together the longer the duration of experience: the fewer bursts, the briefer the overall experience. There must be a space between one pulse of light and the next by definition. Making reference to the breath of our lives and of the cosmos, the Essenes reminded that "in the moment betwixt the breathing in and the breathing out is hidden all mysteries..." The spaces between quantum bursts may be viewed as small expressions of the stillness between each breath. In the silence between the pulses of creation, in the spaces Between, we have the opportunity to 'jump' from one possibility to the next. This space is where the miracles occur.

In <u>Limitless Mind</u>, Russell Targ concludes his Preface saying, "The data from remote viewing research show, without a doubt, that our mind is limitless and that our awareness both fills and transcends our ordinary under-standing of space and time. Psychic abilities, and remote viewing in particular, point to the possibility of our residing in - and as - this state of expanded, timeless, fearless, spacious awareness. Psychic abilities are neither sacred nor secular; they are just natural human abilities. We can use them to find lost keys or elusive parking spaces, to forecast changes in the stock market, or to discover who we really are. I believe that 99 percent of the value of psychic abilities resides in the opportunity they offer for self-inquiry and self-realization. Let's see if we can accomplish this together."

"A philosophic concept isn't necessary to learn and improve, provided a fixed process or ritual is present. **In the case of remote viewing, the scientific study of psi functioning, the protocol is the ritual.**"

"The most renowned remote viewer in the United States" (<u>Reader's Digest</u>), **Joseph McMoneagle** - first introduced to me in a one-hour documentary followed by perusal of his book <u>Mind Trek</u> - had a near death experience while in the Army in 1970 which opened him to spontaneous psychic flashes. For twenty years he honed and developed his skills in a top-secret military program (code name STARGATE) developing and refining scientific protocols for information retrieval for national security purposes.

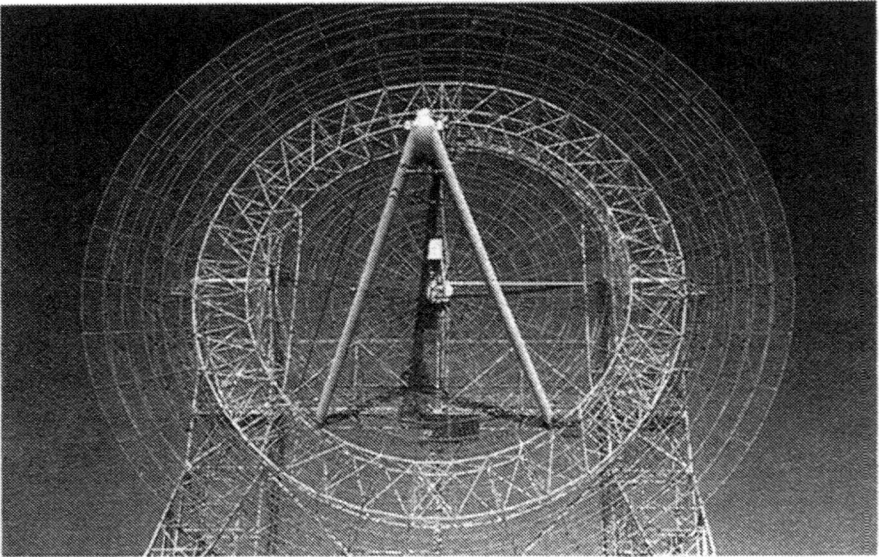

Figure 23. Target Picture in Washington, D.C., Office.

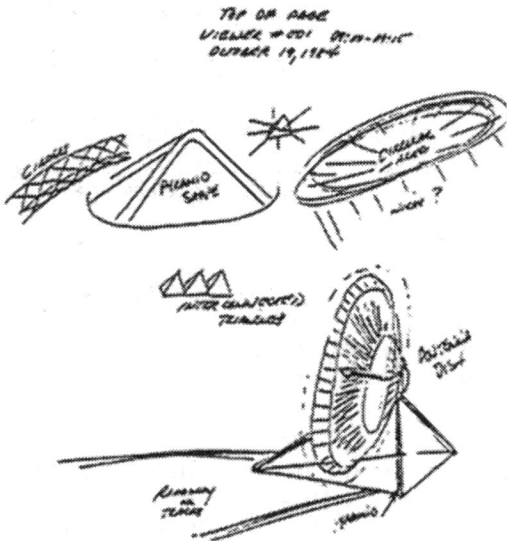

Fig 24. from
Mind Trek
by Joseph McMoneagle

Picture sealed in envelope by person not-known in MD, placed on table in familiar office in DC and drawn remotely in VA by McMoneagle, then faxed to DC

He reports that, starting with "**a temporary suspension of disbelief**" creating a temporary *mysticism*, that he would also call creativity or imagination, after 3 years of remote viewing he had suspended his own disbelief so many times that he was stuck aground somewhere between the *I believe* and the *I know*. He then went through an emergence "which might be considered religious in nature". "Once you've gone through a door and viewed the other side, it's more difficult of not impossible to forget what you've seen or experienced. So backing away from a new reality is a choice that must be taken before you go through the door, not after." He found that, "When you alter one side or perspective, you must change the counter side as well." "What had actually happened was quite simple. Through no deliberate effort, I modified a sufficient number of personal realities or concepts, to unhinge my understanding of time/space, or at least the way I had been originally taught and understood it to work."

Arriving at this place of understanding about self and other, with out-of-body experiences increasing since the beginning of remote viewing training, when he was developing good - if not *knowing* - proficiency, he began to have *other* experiences. These he called *flashes of spontaneous knowledge* - small bits of data that would jump into his mind when he wasn't expecting it. "Perhaps when I would touch objects or people. It wasn't something that I wanted to happen; it just did. At first I would just write it down in my notebook and then forget about it, but then after a while, [reviewing the notebook] I would begin to notice that I was getting *feedback* … important here because it probably has a great deal to do with the transmittal of psychic information. How or why it works I don't know, but it does." Over time he found that wrong information in that stream was *wrong* because it was more of a conclusion than a statement of fact. He "understood early on that the information is usually accurate; what we do with it, how we interpret it, usually isn't." As he improved his observations of the bits and pieces of data that had no relationship to what he was experiencing, "coming to fewer conclusions and recording it as clearly and as cleanly as it actually came to me, I began to see interesting connections to later happen-ings. It was as if I were beginning to grasp how to control the input." The déjà vu experience most entities have had is getting the feedback before something actually happens.

"Perhaps that is what psychic functioning is - a closed loop. We are simply sending ourselves the information which we will know at some future date anyway." This sense of witness and 'opening your mind a mite' just described - recording spontaneous feedback to find a pattern - can be a useful technique for the writer or the reader to adopt in exploring the psi realm (just don't go too far, or nothing here will feel the same).

At this point, I want to interject some echoing admonitions from Seth that I just transcribed upon re-viewing the only movie of Jane Roberts channeling that entity, who initially just dictated books to her. Her beginning advice included "opening your mind a mite - in the middle of your ordinary pursuits" Seth thereafter continued, "You may find yourself with a random thought that does not fit in with what you are doing or thinking at the time It seems random because it does not appear to fit in with your organized picture of reality, but it is an important mosaic that you throw away…. I am challenging you to become more and more aware of your waking experience and of those stray thoughts that come "like thieves in the night". They are not official and you don't accept them. Listen to those thoughts. Open your mind a mite further in your ordinary waking life in the middle of your ordinary pursuits and see what miracles are there - and I say Miracles. Miracles because they can hereby (sic) transform your own understanding and your own reality and you have been blind to them because you feel you will lose your identity. Be gentle with your own experience! Do not be such a disciplinarian that, when stray thoughts or intuitions come to you, you dismiss them."

"The eyes together, being themselves, see for you. The atoms within these eyes do not see this image, though **you** do. You interpret the image [edited down to 10% by the Thalamus] and see what you see. So there is no discipline between your official reality and those unofficial realities that sometimes peek (seek?) through."

*The Seth Video, made by Richard Kendall and Jane Roberts' hus-band Robert F Butts in 1986, is the only visual record we have for these transmissions. There are many books and those about Over-soul Seven provided for me a viable idea about my entity continu-ance, indicating that this discrete part of All-There-Is probably won't continue after leaving these dimensions, but could rejoin a soul group to evaluate the trip and decide on future incarnational ventures.

Joseph McMoneagle began to have spontaneous lucid dreams "with astounding regularity". I have explored this area and wrote a chapter on my experiences with lucid dreaming in **Edgehouse - Embracing the Energies of Change**. Being mentally alert and aware after Joseph realized in the middle of a dream that he was sleeping "was an exceptionally good place in which the imagination could operate. Therefore… also an exceptional area for the subconscious to communicate with the conscious mind, It was the ultimate theater or playhouse." Unfortunately he found that, though he was able to create scenarios of clarity where his subconscious could communicate what it needed to, without conscious mental overlay or interference, the information improved, but the translation or interpretation didn't." He was still subject to human necessity that required conclusions, interpretations, and linear reality construct. "Since the old realities weren't allowing improvement, I began to search for new concepts."

Concepts from the *I believe* column have to be replaced, i.e. unlearned, for the concept's other side to appear in the *I know* column of experience. "Concepts of how reality works are important to remote viewing because they have a direct bearing on where the information comes from and how it might be getting to the remote viewer. They also affect the allowances that might be made within the viewer's mind, the degree of temporary suspension of disbelief, or how far a viewer is willing to go in order to accomplish psychic functioning." **One of the first exceptions to the established rule that goes out the reality window is that there is a difference between past, present, and future information.** In the beginning the remote viewer believes all three types are different and not quite equally accessible. In the beginning, one collects information from real time targets and assumes the information to be fixed in time/space in order to target it. But that begins to fall apart, because, **"once you accept real-time psychic functioning as possible, you automatically begin to violate the assumption of fixed information."** Over the years Joseph has come to know as truth that "Quantum waves do travel in both directions through time. Therefore, in the fullest sense of the word, existence becomes a sum of all information. Like a great sea with far reaching shores. There is no past, no present, and no future - there just *is*. To define our place within it we require a tool some call **cognitive perception.**"

"**Perception** is a process that allows us to place ourselves within a specific point in time and space by observation; **cognition** allows us to understand its dimensions. In simpler terms, we collect information from the past and the future, combine it with what we have in a temporary historical reference (or what we call memory), and **our minds then tells us where and when we are**. Being psychic is simply being more sensitive to the sea around us. It's simply a method that allows for additional sense of being. "Such concepts seemed to seriously modify and/or attack or destroy basic beliefs regarding such subjects as predestination, free will, and God's influence - implying fixed futures, parallel universes, and an overall grand design, and seeming to do away with innovative or changing possibilities." Over time, Joseph has come to understand that "the effect is actually quite the opposite", with the concepts reinforcing his understanding of what free will means and expanding his "concepts of the great engineer we call God. In shorter terms, I now have an even greater miracle to ponder."

"In our desire to seek time travel, we have failed to understand that we are the ultimate time machine. Our consciousness is one with and part of the sea, and through the process called life we pick the space and place in time in which we desire to participate, to exist. Through the tools of perception and cognition, we mold and shape our concept of reality and make reality what it is."

Somewhere along his path, one other significant change became apparent to Joseph. Somewhere in the experiences that were going on in his reality, he stopped caring about proving anything to anyone. He suddenly acknowledged that he knew remote viewing worked, psi-functioning worked, in fact, he expected it to. "So, many of my older concepts of time and space simply withered on the vine and died. The path of my adventure had changed direction, and there was a new horizon to face."

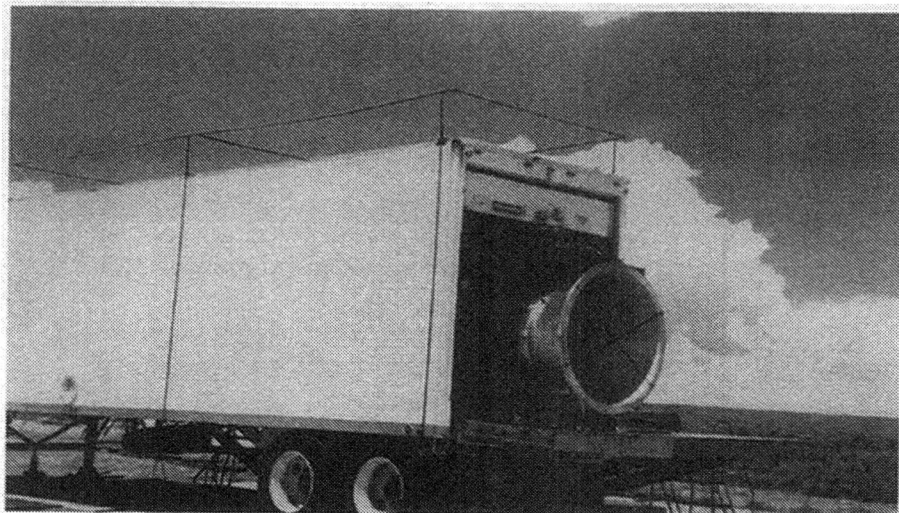

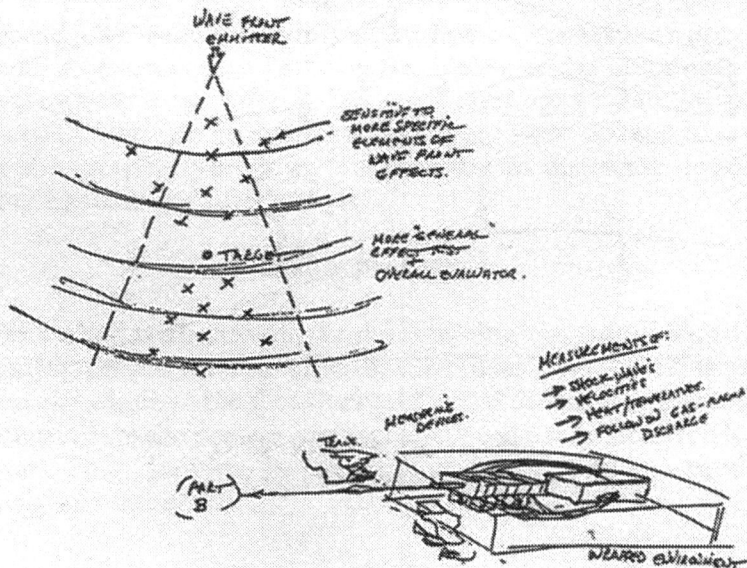

Microwave Generator (Courtesy of CSL)

Example Two
(The microwave generator previously noted by Dr. Jessica Utts.)

I was shown the photograph of an unknown individual and told that he was currently working on a technical site somewhere in the Continental United States. I was asked to describe what he was working on.

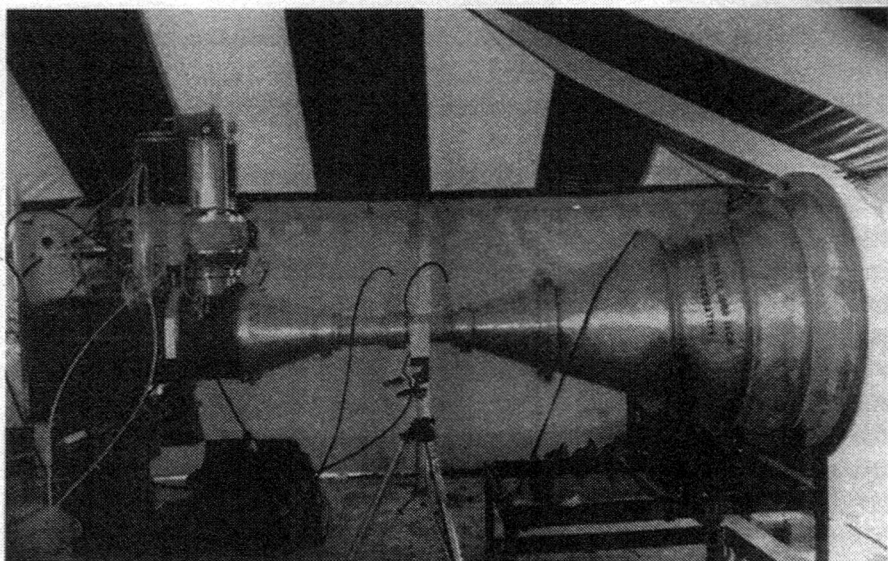

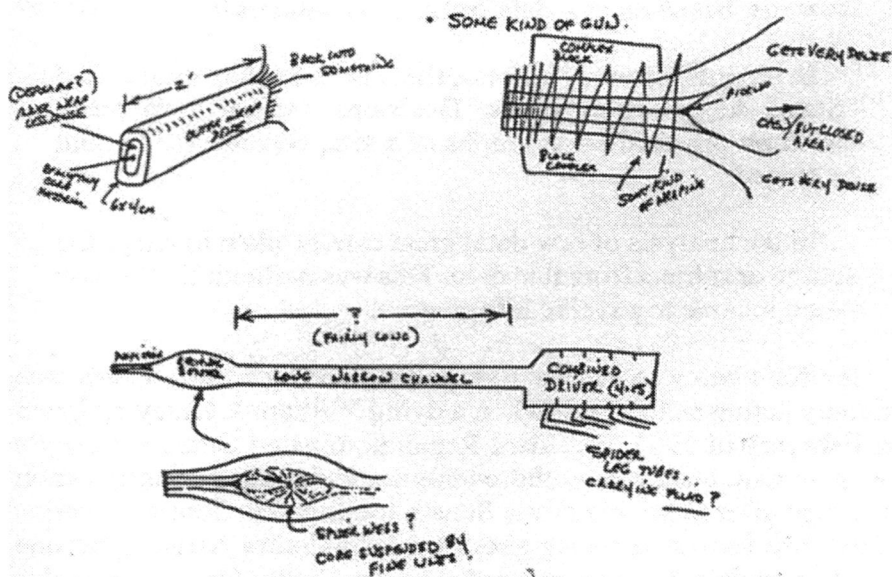

Microwave Generator (Courtesy of CSL)

I found that Example Two operates on a 5 cycle bass wave ELF. Bell Labs partnered with the French to create a van-located device for crown control that looks like a big stadium loudspeaker. Opening the doors pointing the van at the crowd makes everyone drop to their knees with stomach nausea, In <u>Mind Trek</u>, Joseph did not report what he thought about Example Two, but you do remember that suspending judgement is an important part of the Protocol of Remote Viewing.

PERSONAL REMOTE and

not so remote VIEWING

In 1976, at the conclusion of a course in **Silva Mind Control** (then called 'Alpha Awareness' out of justifiable squeamishness over the idea of controlling minds), I quite unexpectedly came to know **personal remote viewing**. Like **Arica**, another school of meditative access to the realm beyond normal consciousness also taught at that time at the Amherst (MA growth) Center, seekers used a simple count-down breathing technique to access and maintain an interactive meditative state in which they were coached over some time by teacher or partners to build a psychic laboratory somewhere in their minds, which is presumed to be located in the head. With Silva, we painstakingly sculpted a big chair or throne in that mind space with a table in front of it. With Arica, the seeker also provided two wall ports in the mental space, through which mother or father, later others, were drawn to the table for examination.

Three-dimensional visualization is where I work and lurk as an artist and designer, so I sculpted a grand throne seat in my mind space from a very large tree. I gave less attention to the table and surrounds. On the final day, working with a partner in my meditation I was given a name and a birthdate of someone unknown to me to examine that she read from one side of a 3 x 5 card. I considered him on my table and noted and reported out three things - a large hole through his left abdomen, 6 - 8 stacked children's wooden blocks with letters on them instead of a neck, and a claw-like right hand. Emerging from meditation, we turned the card over to find this to be a man who had had a major car accident and lost his left kidney. His spinal nerves were *blocked* by a broken neck and the tendons of his right forearm severed, causing an inwardly cramped hand.

My career as Registrar at the time involved designing all the first-time computer systems for student records at

UMass (IBM knew nothing about higher education). My expression then of this abrupt rearrangement of my belief system was that it had "tilted my computer", a meaningless phrase for opening a hole in consciousness today. A new and unshatterable paradigm had been introduced to me, however, now proven to be *remote viewing,* which had given me a glimpse of the All-That-Is that has provided me with **an immutable *knowing*.**

Alpha training teaches people to work in the 7-14 Hz range, which seems to open up psi abilities. Dr Ross Adey's research indicates that 6-20 Hz frequency is needed for the brain neuronal calcium efflux events, with maximum stimulation at 16 Hz. Using a 450 MHz microwave carrier-wave amplitude modulated by an ELF of 16 Hz, he found that ElectroMagnetic fields and the EM mantle around our bodies affect brain function and short- and long-term potentiation of the neurones with a concomitant affect on memory. [Mind control, weather control, inter-dimensional time and travel operations extensively use *and modulate* a carrier transmission wavelength of 435 MHz.] 'Normal' people, entrained to function at high Beta above the 20 Hz threshold, have no contact with neuronal calcium efflux events. If these events are, as he believes, an integral part of Remote Viewing and other psi operations, the general Beta public will be psi-damped, not exhibiting para-psychological talents to any marked degree.

Major Ed Dames (Retired) has stated that military remote-viewers operate in the Theta brain wave frequencies of 4-7 Hz, probably more powerful for psi activity**. If we lower the frequency of our brainwaves we can think with less energy and our biophysical remote-viewing vehicles are therefore more efficient.**

A **second psi glimpse,** more recent for me, has been learning the **protocol** to access wavelengths beyond the edge of normal perception manifest as **auras** - to *know* of this physical dimension from personal experience as **Pranic Healing, a state of being found at the edge of perception, where other psi dimensions are found. Well known, is that the physical body is surrounded by a mantle of electromagnetic energy - a bioelectric field which acts like a blueprint of the physical body.**

At the same time, this mantle of energy supplies us electro-magnetically with the required life energy, rather like a battery. This force can be photographed or scanned with appropriate equipment. Our vitality depends on the size of this force field, and when evenly distributed around the body, we are in good health. Any blocks or deficiencies in this field will eventually manifest themselves as weakness or disease. Pranic healing involves sensing that mantle of energy at its source in its full extension and electro-magnetically participating in its restorative flow.

The eyes pick up the photonic aspects of this energy emission, though 90% of this information is filtered out by the Thalamus, with what comes through the transmission fitted into a visual-mental model which we indeed perceive as reality. Once this visual perception can be unfiltered, auras can be seen around people by some.

The **pacemaker** or rhythm section of the brain is located deep within the brain in the **thalamus**. Calcium ions slowly leak into single thalamocortical neurons which oscillate for 1.5-28 seconds triggering and entraining the brain waves which spread upwards throughout the brain. With excess calcium build-up a 'silent phase' lasting from 5 to 25 seconds yields the brainwaves to be **susceptible to entrainment by external fields**. The electroencephalographic waves spread not only throughout the brain, but through the nervous system via the perineural system into every part of the organism. In this way, brainwaves regulate the overall sensitivity and activity of the entire nervous system.

In the internal pathways involved in the body's response to external magnetic rhythms, **the pineal gland is the primary magnetoreceptor.** Between 20 and 30% of pineal cells are magnetically sensitive. Various animal tissues contain particles of organic magnetite. There is evidence that geomagnetic pulsations strongly entrain brain waves during meditation and other practices in which one 'quiets the mind' to allow the 'free run' to be dominated by geophysical rhythm. The Schumann resonance of earth, thousands of times stronger than brain waves, conducted throughout the body by the perineural and vascular systems can take over as a pacemaker.

The biomagnetic field projected by the hands and coursing through the body can be much stronger than brainwaves indicating that an amplification of at least 1000 times takes place somewhere in the body. Alternatively, the body may simply act as an effective antenna or channel for the Schumann micropulsations. **Schumann waves pulsing between earth and the ionosphere have been generated from the beginning by NASA in order for humans whose brains are entrained to them to live in space**.

The frequent recollection of those who have come through a serious accident or life threatening situation is of time seeming to slow down – an altered perception of time and space. The experience of time slowing down is probably caused by a speeding up of the thalamic clock or pacemaker so that each second is divided into more conscious units. While perceived as a slowing of time it is actually a speeding up of the microgeny – the steps in the processing of data – allowing for more rapid responsiveness needed to initiate life-saving actions.

The high basal stress levels of Western man, releasing torrents of neurohormonal and electrical stimuli, appear to switch off the inherent psi genes. Instead, this over-stimulation seems to switch on the oncogenes that cause cancer. Paranormal abilities are rare in the general population. It is necessary to learn new mental software to switch on the psi genes, lowering stress and over-stimulation. **Paranormal abilities will invariably open up by learning and practicing a protocol of techniques that have provided an undeniable knowing**. Habitual relaxation and mental silence, clearing the mind by focussing directed attention, can switch on latent remote viewing and psi abilities.

In the case of auric energy manipulation, **the psi access protocol involves pranic breathing,** which on the surface greatly slows down the tide of the breath, changes oxygen, nitrogen, and carbon dioxide components of the blood, and confounds the involuntary mechanisms regulating breathing. The hands are sensitized by this protocol beyond their usual boundaries and, lo and bebold, they can receive and send wavelengths probably located just beyond the perceptual edge of what is interacted with as heat. The hands become both receivers and transmitters of body energy, unconsciously yet somehow oh-so-precisely cupped and focussing they facilitate an interchange of now-perceivable wave-lengths of the vibration of living. One learns through the protocol to sense the arms from the elbows down as entirely different appendages in sync with flowing and aware body energies. As in remote viewing, **intention** is the key conceptual access state. Joseph McMoneagle says, **"Intention is the glue that holds everything together.** All of reality as we know it exists because we intend it to. I suspect that if we didn't intend it to be, then it wouldn't." Perceiving and moving auric energy is more than imagination, more than belief - it is as real as anything of living can be. It is a province of psychic healing that for beginners is especially dramatic when working to heal one's self, because the energy can be very precisely felt and moved around deep within the body - when the hands are 5 - 8 inches away from it - clothes on or clothes off. Eventually, as *intention* becomes familiar, without the hands.

Pranic healing teaches practitioners to tactually scan and feel disturbances in the energy body, detecting energetic blockage and *congestion* or energetic deficiency or *depletion*. It works with meridian energy, but unlike acupuncture, Pranic Healing concentrates on the largest meridians, along which the major chakras lie. Pranic Healing is an external-generation system wherein students are taught powerful techniques of breathing and *intention* that enable them to draw in energy from outside the body and then project it into areas of deficiency for healing.   Your energetic anatomy, energy body, or aura is a 3D cloud of prana that begins inside the body in 11 major chakras and a network of light meridians, and emanates outward in all directions to form a rough and somewhat varying outline around your body.

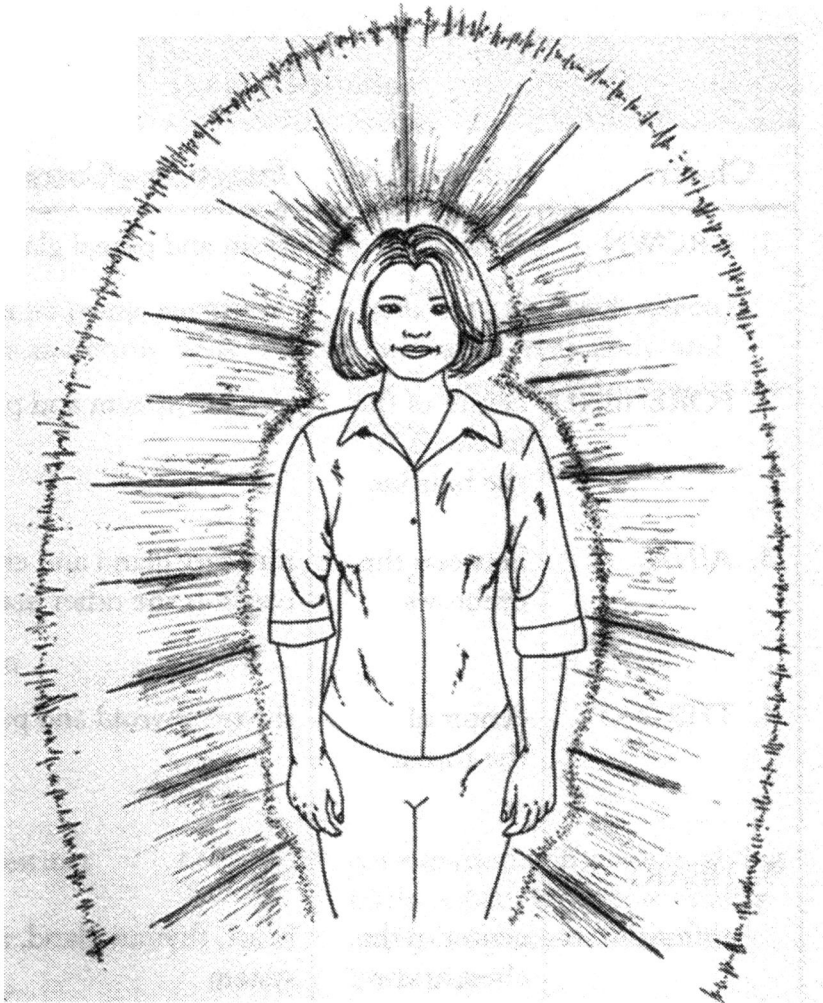

The **inner aura** begins inside the body and extends about 5" out of the body in a healthy adult. The **outer aura** extends up to several feet beyond the inner aura and holds in the body's energy. The **health aura** is an aggregate of 2-ft long beams or rays that radiate from the body's pores - straight and well defined in health, crooked in sickness.

There are 3 principle prana sources - **air prana**, absorbed unconsciously in the act of respiration, **solar prana** from exposure to sunlight, and **ground prana** absorbed through our walking feet (food is an indirect way of absorbing air, earth, and sun prana). **The root cause of energetic disturbances is frequently negative thoughts and emotions, which manifest in the energy body before becoming apparent in the physical body**.

Healing occurs in the energy body before it becomes apparent in the physical body as well. Certainly your health can be affected by external factors such as bacteria and viruses, poor life choices, bad habits, and accidents, but illness may result from energetic disturbance that is at root caused by the unconscious mind trapping negative emotion or limiting belief in the body

'Inspire' means to draw in spirit: 'expiring' is breathing out the life force. **Pranic breathing** is diaphragmatic or full abdominal breathing through the nose and expanding the tension-holding abdominal muscles under the rib cage up and to the front and the sides, with the subtly sinuous spine arching back to maximally pull down the diaphragm and to draw air deeper through the top two-thirds of the lungs into the bottom third, providing a richer flow of oxygenated blood and prana, as well as providing muscular movement to pump the cleansing lymphatic system. The exhale through the nose can be imaged as an unforced arching forwards of the whole spine to the top of the head, relaxation of the abdominal extension and space, with the spine bowing forward and the chest lifting such that <u>a sine wave of the spine is provided in each extended breathing of a prana cycle</u>. Another bowed-forwards full retention pause of air prana body self-awareness **image**, has the extension of that **inspiration** of pranic energy with consciousness eventually flowing upwards from the expanded bowels along the spine behind the lungs and reaching the throat - even the crown - then spilling out on the exhale. **By lifting/opening the chest on both the inhale and the exhale, the spine augments the bellows of breathing. In this way of following the breath you learn to feel and move your consciousness around with the energies within the body.**

The concept of 'image' denotes a mental activation of all the muscles involved in a given stance in opposition to or in conformity with the influences of gravity, and an awareness of all of their inter-relatedness and the interactions of muscle and bone without any movement being called for. Enthralled in the activated image of self, arching back on exhale (mid spine forward) and forward on inhale (mid spine back) without physical movement, I call this **isometric yoga**. [I dove inside with pranic breathing recently during 3 hours' captivity in an airplane, and I full-bodied danced to the classical head-set sound stream for over 2 hours - feeling all of the different places on my stockinged feet that touched earth with different dance movements - joyously twitching ever so imperceptably - grinning in my seat, and eventually perspiring. My 'dancing' was interrupted by CBS - I mean a stewardess who works for CBS, I mean United, but then the same 2 hours of CBS ads I had already been subject to the last 2 flights seemed predictable as the corridors of Dulles bore CBS also emblazoned ... what happened? The new gay LOGO channel even has "CBS News" spots)(ok, I was way out there)

The pranic breathing rhythm also performs the same protocol function as chanting or repetition of a mantra in focussing the attention. The energy-producing capacity is increased ten-fold when retention at the end of each cycle is extended. **Holding the breath after each exhalation is *empty retention*, creating a powerful physiological and energetic vacuum.** Holding after inhalation is *full retention*, together creating a pranic 'bellows effect', magnifying prana's natural cleansing and energizing affects on controlled exhale to reach more fully and easily into the cells, organs, and chakras within your body.

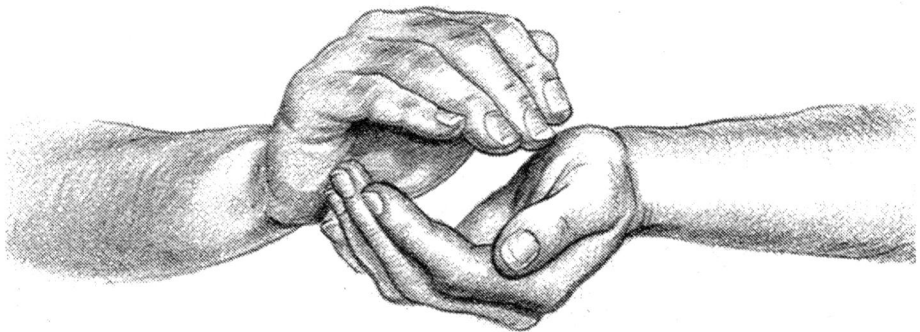

The aura around the body varies somewhat from day to day and, in the protocol also, after energizing the hands with several repetitive extended arm and snapping exercises and after feeling the palms slowly tranform. They come alive to their transition into sensing, emitting, and receiving; feeling the embodiment of two **transducers**, a new but somehow familiar thing/awareness to have at the ends of your arms enters. With reactivated hands one first tests and visually measures the distance of the becoming-ever-more-familiar auric energy 'layer' that is most easy to perceive through one's focussed *intention* at several points like hips, knees, head and neck. Slowly swinging the activated more and more mirroring moving arms and hands in towards the body, I sometimes sense an encasing body sheath at about 18" away, but with my *intention* fully in place, initially at around 5" on the sides and 8" in front of the pelvis, the hands encounter a more tangible layer that can be stroked or clawed, with clear precisely-matching surface or indeed internal body perception of the interaction. Focussing the hands extremely precisely on myself, yet without any interfering thought about it, I work on the prostate, pelvic girdle around to the back, specific internal organs that can be sensed in detail where the consciousness moves without hesitation, and on the kundalini blockages in the neck.

Working to channel the ever more perceptible flow of energy that you can transduce in the joyful process of your own healing provides body feed-back allowing you to more quickly recognize and claim the difference between the 'willing' and the 'intending' entity states of mental and body consciousness. When that feeling that one previously described as warmth, or was it cold, comes on to the edges of the loosely cupped hand, usually for me the heel is first followed by the curved thumb column. The energy sensation is vividly ambivalent. You are conscious of three things. When the hand is connected in to this band of wavelength auric light, seemingly not seen behind the brain-filtered vision, it feels in itself, more on the surface, a flow that is circulating and noticeably charging the body. Much of the time in daily life clasped, one's hands usually close this circuit to promote an embedded resonance. I would call what the hands of *intention* now feel *'transduceing'* - sensing, indeed hastening, that flow that is circulating throughout all and charging the body. All mental programming controlling the hands' shaping as dish antennae with focus, or as emitting fingers with energy, is turned back to sub-autopilot. Those hundreds of muscles and bone articulations know precisely their antenna function and conscious mind is an interference. They can focus around in back of you all precisely skewed OR on any convenient location you can **intend** them and you can then follow their energy most precisely within.

This focus is so far somewhat exhausting after a half an hour or so - faintly aerobic somehow. The re-alignment of my body energies is noted by clicks and abrupt shifts in muscle-bound joint orientations. My early pranic breathing had a lumbar click and release accompanying each oh-so-languid breath. Startling is, when working from neck to occiput with the focussed hand-power beam and all over the skull (advisedly avoiding the eyes), several skull bones click into hopefully more energy-efficient adaption, as the neck already has, including even some inner ear clicks of readjustment. It's still a very new extension of psi abilities for me, but it is as real as can be and I know I will venture further with my *intention* to explore this especial psi ability, affecting the health of my body and hopefully eventually the bodies of other people for healing.

I'm beginning to wonder about **other healing**, though, as the hands close some sort of *intention* circuit with specific loci within my body, yet the hands can eventually be mostly defused though remaining available, while the hurtsogood focus continues its guiding healing path within.

You could say this whole self-deception (instead of *'intention'*) is just heat perception. I'll accept that, because what is heat but a perceived band of energy wavelengths that all things living and inert objects as well emit and receive at all times in this consensual dimensional grid? I exult in the opening of myself at the very edges of my perception as I think you do too.

Finding an energic center as a playing field consciousness grid to access the other intentions to interact with the All-That-Is may not deviate far from that old 'witness' concept that I was earlier promoting for myself. It is less ambitious as a realizing entity, it is true. It's a little more entity-based, while abandoning contact with what's believed to be 'out there' for immersion 'in here'. Sort of saying 'good luck' to the out-there-in-empty-space not involved with my current body incarnation script. My adopted generation was 'for' 'getting down'. Still connected with pot, somehow - it works for me to access the fringes of my physical personality - the edges of the **con**[jobof]**science** [how'd that get in there?].

When working with auras, I have scene that restoring visual perception and observing while energized hands detect, run up against, and interact with the body on an auric level does not deactivate those hands - it does so only if I evaluate or judge what I think I see. *Intention* rules.

INTENTION, NOT IN TENSION

I'm opposed to tension in a relaxed way. Especially in the body. Giving up body tension is ever more important to revving up self-healing. This past year I have focused my *intention* on learning to activate and fully sense transducing *handtenna* through *protocol* and I have come to locating and moving energy throughout the body on *intention* with or without the hands, to my continual *mirth*. Your body will do whatever your mind intends – just bypass the internal evaluative dialog and know and realize your *intention*.

My sculptor's hands led to this another major modification in my belief system. I have appreciated even followed as it were a half dozen gurus and spiritual disciplines from the 70s-on who did teach focus, but. Maybe vipassana had you steering your mind about in the body and looking for places needing attention and repair, but there was no dialog about going there <u>right now</u> and interceding - other than 'chanting' reinforcing affirmations or by joining your energy with for-profit groups, usually run by come-lately seekers who were still searching.

The body is, throughout, in a form of constant tension and compression - being pushed down by gravity and from its own unique upright interactions and ontogeny. When the tensions between the energies of the body's diverse movement and support systems can be *fully relaxed in a way they never are*, those systems can participate in overt and overall body vibrations as suggested by years of exploring bioenergetics. The wavelengths/frequency of those waves while standing (though it is quite possible to exercise them from most postures) can be nodally controlled in frequency by where consciousness is placed and moved. The waves seem to originate with consciousness pressing down or with calculated grounding around the balls of the feet.

When I first extended the standing wave, that connects somehow to adolescent male's restless legs and is fairly accessible, to include shoulders and then sustainedly 'snapped' the neck beyond the shoulders in the full-body sinusoidal beat, I was intrigued by the clicking of the occiput/atlas spine top as well as the rippling spine itself (which doesn't click any more unless startled). Discovering that the fully relaxed body would participate at different faster beats based on contact support nodes when leaning back and seated on furniture, next obvious was to consciously play these chords of nodal cooperation and get down into some real vibrations of living.

A standing body wave has very specific nodal locations and the wavelength is pitched by *intention*. Sometime after the body wave has embodied and with physical adjustment scanning to reorient, sometimes painfully especially in the neck, the conscious body so that its energy fields come into alignment, specific body energy locations are identified and assumed as body focus of available consciousness not really distracting from the wavelength of standing expression of the energy-amalgam that an entity has summoned with *intention* to this day in our time. **These loci I call nodes and their location in the larger wave form determines its frequency.** You consciously move (slide?) the more central nodes until a new sinospinal wave length expresses a most distinct change. This is aTuning.

The protocol of Master Co was just the right beginning for me to pop open new dimensions of selfing, self-actively pursued since the 60s. Changing the over-all body balance and energy flow and the sensate ions of the hands to establish points of consciousness transfer within the body's auric field is the *intentional* tool of this successful quest for focus and an altered state reality. One's awareness accepts that very much different hands become alternate appendages (from the elbows to infinity, it seems to me) that are focusers, perhaps projectors, of the *intention*. Operating at almost any distance when contact with internal consciousness points or areas is made, they are simply projections of your *intention* and any adjustment of their no-more-under-motor-control beam maintenance is turned over to your *intent*, away from survival and pleasure instincts. When you learn the energy needs of where-ever your *intention* visualizes the location of its focus, and that the hands are more a physical part of the *protocol* that can be dispensed with, there you are – deep or shallow within – focused where the hands had directed – or distant. Sometimes you follow your intuition for a map to direct your energy – sometimes your *intention* leads you. **Listening and being guided by the process is pivotal in this adventure of self discovery and healing**.

Half the time in the *protocol,* shutting out all-of-out-there, I am groaning or complaining or exulting and commenting - breathing varies between extended pranic cycles with extended empty retention pauses to fast breathing, when, usually pelvic, but all vibrations become aerobic. If I see my expression in the mirror that reflects somewhat the minute-appearing and changing frequency foot to cranium vibrations but doesn't show where my consciousness is focused within, it is slack open and not projecting the visage carapace I usually wear for other entities to see.

You know how you can shift your consciousness right to a cramp or a muscle complaint? Or how you have learned to move your consciousness very specifically to that certain place within which provides urine release? Well, **this is just going without a doubt (with *intention*) to a specific place within without such a summons.** You could interpret such a focus as pain, as usual, or you can *re-intend* it into a flood of healing *intention* that just hurts to give consciousness to. Standing or sitting vibrationally body stacked, after inhabiting my body with a few adjustments in consciousness, I can clearly feel the suppressed stance and balance of rutting, thrusting, and explore how all those involved energy systems clinging to the rim of the pelvis, gyrating the vestigial tail coccyx (only clockwise, with the Sufis) following and stroking bundled bands of inner thigh muscle, awareness in balls, bouncing demurely. It isn't about sexuality at all, though, but about the complexes of emotional and physical intricacy that have laid down in these energies a holograph of your emotional adjustment to incarnation (well, some of it could be thought of as physical, if you are into that sort of thing).

Coralling your *intention* to focus and feed back the energy situation within, starting with one or two bilateral points deep within, for what will be a possibly prolonged perambulation between your body's energy systems – vibrating to their healing those muscle, nerve, bone and chakral energies emanating from your very own *intention*, entity, is a whole new dimension of *knowing*. A *protocol* is probably initially necessary, especially if you haven't spent alternative time, perhaps with the herb that is my 40-year guide, coming to experience your body without the burden of sexual drives and fantasies that have placed a number of icons on each of our altars of need and desire and insistently but decreasingly with age intrude whenever we 'embody'.

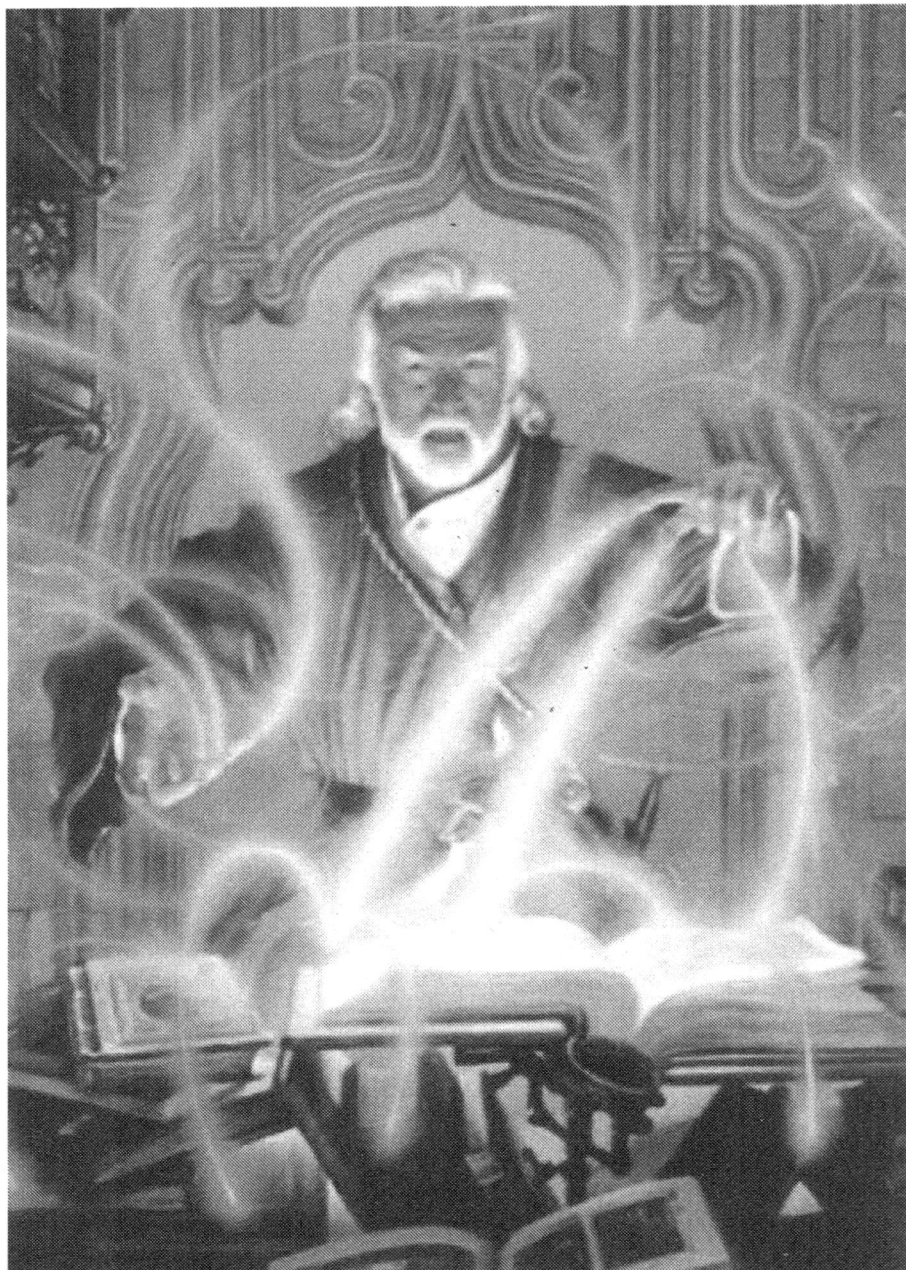

TWO sample EXERCISES

Some of my current healing protocols may illustrate a couple of my perhaps unique *intentions* with embodyment this day in our time. **Here's two sample protocols for opening and relaxing in a way that one never does. And you will *intend* your own:**

I hang from a bar that's just four or so inches below my upwards reach, with feet placed a foot back allowing a fully relaxed pelvic forward thrust pulled open and loose by the up-to-50 lbs at least of lower body pull tension (depending on your relinquishing of support) that **the equalized but variable muscular-bone-pelvis in intimate but tense relationship to both energy directions <u>never</u> experiences** (except in free-fall maybe). With this relaxed interrelatedness and intending and feeling the extension, I gain back the 1 1/2" of height I lost slouching through life. I spend at least five minutes hanging with that extension, giving time to move consciousness in detail to very specific energy locations in the flowing vibrational surgings which really appreciate the attention and make amends.

Alternatively, with feet beyond the bar, relaxed 'unsitting' muscle and sinew complexes savor the unaccustomed energy flow which accompanies my *intentional* consciousness, moving to precisely the points needing and receiving energy healing. In a way, it is the mirror image of tension – relaxed and extended and also present in putting the spine into harmonic vibration when all matched or currently mis-matched energies are intentionally almost fully relaxed. Successive waves of opening receive full consciousness and healing in this daily exercise of extension.

Being treated for lumbar sciatica in 3 adjacent (of course) vertebrae, physical therapy had me bowing and scraping (to free a dorsal disk squeeze at L-3), then arching backwards to deal with an opposite disk compression (L-5). For the last treatment, for the middle centrally-pinched L-4 energy complex, they had me on the rack for 10 minutes at 50 lbs spine-extending pull. This rack I gleefully replicate with this exercise of my afterlife and, under tension of gravity and structural weight, I move consciousness throughout the spine to examine and support it in its late life first exposures to intention's glimpses of freedom from the spinal embodiment that is driven by my unique template of my traumatic stress archives. Moving up spine, those vertaplexes between the threatened-by-hard-heartening shoulder blades absolutely love and crave the experiencing of extension without any tension. Think about it: *hurtsogood* is rampant between the shoulder blades when the bottom falls out.

+++++++++++++++++++++

That spectrum of multiple energies shimmering and variably consciously accessed, named **TASTE**, gives you a chance to *intend* consciousness over that broad spectrum with the absolute knowing of your consciousness' location. **If your *intention* is to have a conscious intimate relationship with the earth prana of your sustenance, you can focus your energy of *intention* into awakening the consciousness of taste into full being**.

When you are aware that you are not focusing your consciousness on your food prana, you must simply take control of your chew beat away from the faithful involuntarily-regulated complex autonomic assimilation program and **simply pause after each chomp**. You also try to control automated swallowing. With your first pause, initial tastes grow and spread immediately by increased saliva and the resistance to swallowing except way back in the mouth. Tastes and awareness blossom and spread in each full pause between chews, which can extend and are disguised meditations of embodiment. After full and extended swallowing, occasional memory savors can usually be found on a mouth search, so don't take on anything else with the old speed and blind intensity. Remember, pauses between each bite. You well know these savors and their trails and the varied mouth locations where each is given due appreciation. Keep pausing and tasting in the various realms of your mouth and control of swallowing will assuredly be with your *intention*. With some foods already in a manna-like liquid/solidarity state, controlled swallowing spread in the back of the mouth region like a vast gustatory oasis, where these states seem to be more appreciated, may accompany every multi-colored and toned evaluative conscious *intention* to 'be there' tasting (as the guy said).

When I notice that I am not paying consciousness to eating (I haven't committed full attention to only eating), a dozen or more times a gustatory day I give my full *intention* a chance to taste, in order to be doing this eating-meeting.

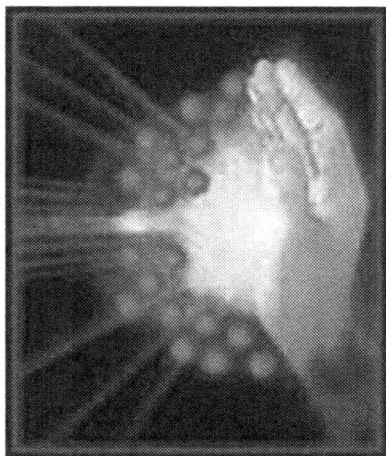

A comprehensive manual on the protocol and practice of Pranic Healing is **Your Hands Can Heal You** by Master Stephen Co and Eric B Robins MD

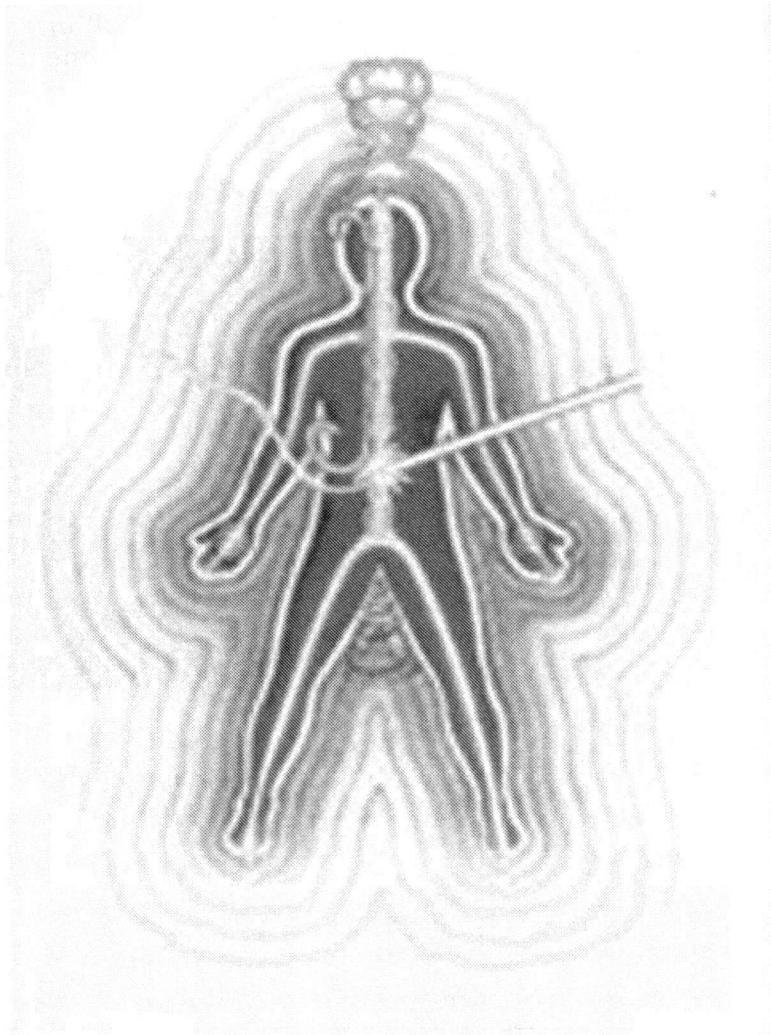

Invitation to the Dance

Israel Regardie (who was Aliester Crowley's secretary 1928-1932 while I was getting born) wrote in his <u>The True Art of Healing</u> about the psi world and "a force which directs and controls the entire course of life that, properly used *(a phrase that could be an illuminati warning)*, can heal every affliction and ailment to which mankind is heir." "By turning the fiery penetrating power of the mind inwards upon itself, and exalting the emotional system to a certain pitch, we may become aware of previously unsuspected currents of force. Currents, moreover, almost electric in their interior sensation, healing and integrative in their affect."

"Nothing in the vast expanse of space is dead. Everything pulses with vibrant life."

"The atom is a crystallization of its power."

"How can there be a depletion if vitality and cosmic currents of force daily pour through man, simply saturating his mind and body [*entrained in Schumann waves, absolutely*) with its power? Primarily it is because he offers much resistance to its flow through him that he becomes tired and ill, the conflict finally culminating in death. The complacency and confusion of his mental outlook, the moral cowardice by which he was reared, and his false perception of the nature of life – these are causes of resistance to the inward flow of spirit." "Man surrounds himself with a crystallized shell of prejudice and ill-conceived fantasies, an armor which affords no entrance to light of life without."

"The first step towards freedom and health is conscious realization of the vast spiritual reservoir in which we live and move and have our being." "The second step towards freedom lies in a slightly different direction. Regulated breathing – quite a simple process. It's necessity follows from the following postulate. If life is – all about one, all penetrating and all pervasive, what is more reasonable than that the very air we breathe from one moment to another should be highly charged with vitality? Our breathing processes we therefore regulate accordingly. We contemplate that life is the active principle in the atmosphere."

"It is fundamental and important that the initial rhythm (of taking in air prana) should be maintained, for it is that very rhythm itself which is responsible for easy absorption of vitality from without, and the acceleration of the divine power within."

"Cultivate above all the art of relaxation. Learn to address each tensed muscle from toe to head as you lie flat on your back in bed [or even stand or sit]. Tell it deliberately to loosen its tension and cease from its unconscious contracture. Think of the blood in response to your command flowing copiously to each organ [like a rising and filling tide of the body's energies], carrying life and nourishment everywhere, producing a state of glowing radiant health. Only after these preliminary processes have been accomplished should you begin your rhythmic breathing, slowly and without haste. Gradually as the mind accustoms itself to the idea, the lungs will take up the rhythm spontaneously. In a few minutes it will have become automatic. The whole process then becomes extremely simple and pleasurable."

"It would be impossible to overestimate its importance or efficacy. As the lungs take up the rhythm, automatically inhaling and exhaling to a (newly introduced) measured beat, so do they communicate it and gradually extend it to all the surrounding cells and tissue – just as a stone thrown into a pool sends out widely expanding ripples and concentric circles of motion. In a few minutes the whole body is vibrating in unison with their movement, Every cell seems to vibrate sympathetically (and harmonically). And very soon, the whole organism comes to feel as if it were an inexhaustible storage battery of power. The sensation – and it must be a sensation is unmistakable. Simple as it is, the exercise is not to be despised. It is upon the mastery of this very easy technique that the rest of the system stands. Master it first. Make sure that you can completely relax and then produce the rhythmic breath in a few seconds.

Pranic Healing

   I have come to the realization that my decades of "healing" massage, polarity, acupressure, transferring energy to other entities culminating, I thought, with auric intercession, won't be an *intended* reality for me until my healing – easy to access, to generate, to jump into altered body consciousness/healing with focused *intention*, is Enough. How this I know is that, when those newly/again energized hands initially find a strokable energy film 5 or so inches away from my standing waist, my consciousness recognizes that contact from within the body at the focus of the hand's energies and closes a flowing interactive circuit of *intention* fully sensed by this embodiment alone. Two hands connect with two points of anywhere body consciousness and awareness moveable by spiritophysico appendages at the bidding or dismissal of *intention*, an *intention* that eventually can even do without the hands' apparently necessary circuit closing function in order to focus within, when and where *intention* decides.

   Before *intention* goes all the way, though, the *handtenna* set about their intended task of re-grounding the **instanding** by stroking post traumatic stressed body energy painfully downward from torso out the ends of the toes or into the chakra 9" below the feet. I say painfully, because that is the only sensation available to the perceptual internal nerveworks, familiar in massage for example, and **healing thus hurts so good**. After the body's energy is circuiting, the next 10 minutes or so can be spent moving consciousness at its *hurtsogood* focus at any depth, usually slow speed, following where it and the hands and the *intention* leads, pausing sometimes as the need is felt for longish periods of healing contemplation painfully expressed. Generally at Master Cho's direction, this energy, retrieved from detailed pelvic perusal, is stroked or 'clawed' downward, following/listening to its *intended* suggestions and directions – sometimes down the whole leg and even out, but usually in generated guided waves that need smoothing through the knees and cluster in shins and calves. These energy waves need special attention in order to chase them out of heels and ankles, along insteps and outsteps, 'milking' the foot tops, gently guided out of the toes to Beyond. Sometimes perception of the accumulated de-tired-us seems so jammed up in calves and ankles and the gravity-balancing tendons and 26 bones of each foot that a languid energic slowplow is needed to move it all Out.

Sometimes these pranic cleansing energy sweepings ride a single distended and suspended exhalation into the funset, insistingly demanding emptying-time for re-sweeping, for grouping, extracting, and corralling the recalcitrant *hurtsogood* vestiges down-leg that clearly belong gone with the immanent extension and ultimate roundup of still prana-full don't knead and haven't kneeded breath (sorry, that got away from me).

The activity of exhaling is a learned behavior. It begins early to dominate over natural natal inhaling and exhaling with the onset of fear. Born we are with the inhale taking in life and with gracefull relaxation in the exhale preparing our embodyment for another taste of *prana* (Seth says we are blinking on and off at the atomic level). We gradually condition ourselves and particularly our autonomic programming to use our increasing fears around our survival to accelerate the urgency to exhale in order to inhale (and save the embodyment). This being the way we come to operate, the very extended cycles of the breath *protocol* in pranic breathing are calculated to allow one to re-gain control over the autonomic or automatic breath cycling long enough to override it, without so much of one's consciousness being subservient to its accustomed mastery. Counting to one's self the timing of the exhale and the inhale is used in initial pranic breathing, and pauses are instigated when the lungs are emptied and when they are filled (*empty retention, full retention*).

My counting of the rate of respiration, rather than by time, is at first more a keeping aware of successive directive consciousness bursts to assume control of exhaling. With my *intention*, I slowly exhale a bit then slightly pause in the *intentional* stream, in order to then renew exhaling to another pause, then count thus the next revisiting of the awareness of the sensation of *intentional* exhalation, and observe the sensings of a series of partial exhalations, proceeding thus unthreatened by the usually insistent autonomic order to breathe. Often, after a longer pause at the end of one cycle, without being on autonomic, I forget whether the controls I have in my *intentional* grasp suggest inhalation next or exhalation. This consciously stepped exhale accompanied by a consciousness focused more and more suffused in the body may include my adjacently bringing awareness to a lifting of the chest and a rolling forward of the lumbar spine pressing up on the diaphragm. Sometimes an inhale may overtake the pranic *intention* once in a while, and it is quick and I return to the exhale busyness. The inhale of pranic breathing has the spine opening back and the stomach relaxing out with the chest still lifting. The inhale is *intentionally* slowed and may comfortably also pause repeatedly as prana is being used, with the aim of gradually and repeatedly topping off the absorption of prana, which increases intake. The lower third of the lung capacity is activated. Where the conscious location of the inhalation incrementally moves within the body is recorded by *intention*, sometimes climbing the spine into the neck or out the top of the head. ("breathe into X") **By my experience, this contemplative pranic breathing must be altering the balance of the gasses carried by the blood delivered to the operating system and altering its perceptions and interaction with the reality I create.** This edge of perception is where you argue with yourself as to what reality you are able to create. We are all oh-so-familiar with that internal dialog. With *intention*, you push beyond enslaving consensual reality into *knowing* something of your other inherent dimensions that accompany incarnation in this plane.

Master Cho says to start your energy gathering protocol with several pranic breaths. What happens when you have trained yourself to the *protocol* is that **when the autonomic breath control mechanism is sidestepped with a few very intentional breaths, the breathing co-joins with rising and building waves of body energy and thereafter takes care of itself in an energy integrated way. The empty pause after exhale can then extend tremendously, inhalation can be shallow and intermittent, conscious attention to a breathing protocol becomes unimportant.** Fears of not getting enough air dealt with in childhood when the air had been knocked out of you falling out of a tree or whenever are set aside. The breath is subservient to the *intention*.

An *intentional* image goal of this pranic breath includes a developing awareness of filling the body with energy like liquid filling a vessel. I feel it slowly rise in legs along with vibration and into the torso, extending into shoulders forearms and hands, where newly familiar sensation begins as hands and forearms may gradually deny their grasping function and assume different properties of sensation and reception. *Intention* now shifts to sensing the hands as in a restructured muscle/bone/sinew and venue way, with their sensing ability dealing in a range of wavelengths only available below the elbow by *intention*. I think of their now alternate possible extension as *transducers* of the body's organic energy built-in to focus the body's *intentional* self-healing. My *intention* suffuses the hands and I am consciously aware as they change state – first the heel, then around to the thumb, then a complete surrender of muscular controls in the *handtenna* that now feel, speak, and sense the body energy.

I reach out the balanced partly aware of themselves hands and caress an intended flat vertical auric plane in front of me to test and assure them of their awakened alternate sensitivity and potential, surrounding and suffocating self-doubts with my creative *intention*. Awareness of the changed appendages builds and I am not in a hurry. Master Cho says at this energy juncture to next test these reenergized hands coming in to opposition to each other. In polarity we were told hands had opposite polarity whatever that means. Even though half my day they may be clasped in some sort of grounding, mine can't find each other's auric edges at all, so for me the hands next move for their activation validation to next sense the aura surrounding my body and are not disappointed. When I have confidence in my realized h*andtenna*, I thus test my body's auric covering, bringing the hands that now tangibly feel themselves differently in towards the body near hips, near the knees, near the chest – touching down on the tangible auric sheath and opening my eyes to verify the touch-down's distance, usually initially at around 5" away. For me, marijuana boosts *intention* and disgraces self-doubting. With it's tangible body changes it facilitates for me body awareness, focus, and consciousness.

At this point, I digress from Master Cho's protocol body environment to invite my now fully-sensed body and arms to vibrate as an *intentionally* plucked energy string of diverse and consciously explored wavelengths. The basic standing ventral-dorsal spinal sinusoidal wave is accessed by pressing down from grounded differential points of foot contact and rattles up to the top of spine atlas/occipital junction with each undulation. This vibration of total relaxation, lacking the usual balanced force of opposing always-active muscles and tendons, comes as **an extension of 20 years of bioenergetics**, seen as well in the adolescent male's restless seated legs.

Starting up the standing body wave for me involves consciously pressing the soles of the feet down in order to stand taller than the gravity of my contemporary avoir-du-pois embodyment, and moving intentionally located body consciousness around in some complex sequence of sole touch-down awarenesses that **begin to generate sinusoidal waves in what might be seen as an *intentionally* reclaimed natal stance (why not?).** My right shoulder drops back into balance as my body fills with pranic energy, in spite of its snapped and gone right biceps and rotator cuff sub-scapularis having been only reattached to 5%. Scoliosis recedes, 3 different lumbar-disc-pressed 3,4,5 sciatica tensions relax, and all of the body seems balanced as it might have been before fear. The *instanding* edge is then created by *intentionally* tuning touch-down body vibrational causes and affects until a basic body frequency already well known from each prior *bodyintending* (and confidently predicted for any time of my future I *intend* it) is welcomed. There, I *instand*, and focus on my top vertebral atlas slide/creaking with each wave to lubricate forgotten paths of spinal energy seeking en-lighten-ment (lift off?). Breathing may go from very prolonged exhalation, without autonomic breathing stimulus or panic reminders, to aerobic shallow and fast breath, with a prolonged standing and nodal-consciousness-stipulated body frequency pattern. The aerobic nature of this vibration limits me, astrally justified with a life-long avoiding of aerobic activities tuned by genetic angina tendencies, to about 15 minutes of this body vibrating *intending* that is also aerobic in one session. The vibrating is a variable and shifting component in this form of body healing, however.

The concept I call *instanding* is of the grounded spinal column with its upward filling and flowing vibration including shoulders but not variably energized arms. Mirrored arms may hang loose, be rigidly extended balanced ahead or above, actively being realized as handtenna, or at the same time even taking over the torso's vibration with a rapid upper harmonic of gradually increasing tem-po. Once flowing, *instanding* can be released from its grounding.

A next direction for change is to close the body energy circuit from indentically freed from their usual functional purpose hands to communicate with and influence very specific internal locations of healing directed by these hands, and to listen to the coursing energy to provide for directional movement – sometimes hovering focused on demanding loci, yet eventually sweeping torso and pelvic and leg energy down the limbs and out as Master Cho directs, to be released into a green fire of *intentional* dispersal. As well as standing, this body healing can be accessed sitting, or in a swinging chair which offers more complex interactive vibrations. Seated, the points of contact are grounding nodes of *intention* for auric releasing and cleansing. Extended some in a chair, the upper thighs are a node resting on its edge with the neck a supporting node for a different torso vibrational wavelength with the legs on a different wavelength on the floor or not. With a pivoting swinging chair this multiple vibration takes on overtones to become very complex and that can self-destruct.

One day's circumambulation comes to rimming the pelvic girdle, **stroking hurtsogood pain downward girdlesides into the juncture of instanding**. Carefully gathering the lower spine-to-coccyx broad girdle and the dimpled gluteal energy foci, I am put on pause there. Pauses on energy foci that insist on more attention are also often instructive in modifying your energy *intentional* path. Moving the genital energy that is rooted throughout the pelvis and down the legs, probably preferring the leg muscles sinews and bone articulation of thrusting over just standing there, doesn't involve actual engagement to engorgement, just the *intention* to heal. Engorgement seems triggered non-tactily only by the mind of lust and the nighttime REM pumping system. The activated vibrational body energy wavelengths in movement connected with standing and thrusting don't seem to switch consciousness over to the *intentions* surrounding one's particularly long-agonized-about sexual arousal *protocol* which the body is *knowing* to be a perilous and energy-wasting side shoot.

Intention is partially focused in your inner mind's image of consciousness' location. It is most often for me a mildly outward streaming goldish locus first available in the dark popping screen upon shutting down 80% of my visually confirmed impressions of what's out there. Your consciousness has learned it can outsmart the physical and it proceeds. It will establish circuitry among its parts allowing moving, observing, and interactive and stand-alone locating anywhere within (without may be on hold). It is such that if you introduce your functional image of between your shoulder blades into that golden locus or maybe into the leaf pattern you are timelessly staring at or move it under your right knee-cap directly, the body energy slumbering in those loci will be changed. And the process will probably be in direct harmonic relationship to *hurtsogood* communication and its cruise control.

In another day's *protocol* arousal, working pelvico-genitally, I learned more about focusing and functioning of handtenna. When I was long lost *instanding in basic headrocker* and sorta playing the occipital-atlas spinetop slidation wave by altering the touchdown of my right foot to change the pitch, my yet-uncalled-for hands riding the bigger wave suddenly, with right thumb audibly(!) snapping into handtenna control, activated into a dark field gold cereal bowl catcher's glove and I became much more aware of the hands' transmissional radiance without being able to see their auric energy. They are perceived oh-so-differently.

More and more lately *protocol* is bypassed as I, in altered pranic focus, dialog whynotnow you can skip the protocol knowing you-can-get-there, just-do-it and 'there we have it!'. So when I recovered my altered self's *intention* to disturb the multi-rational sexual energy and embraced genitals in a 16" diameter power handtenna focus (each hand 8" away), they would surprisingly **move significantly from the impact of breeze-free distant auric stroking**. I returned to watching again as the most intense hurtsogood was experienced, however, rooting around to find the balanced and mirrored handtenna 20 inches away from the groin and to the sides. And through this witness, I recalibrated my interpretation of these energies, checking other energy complexes of the body to confirm that, while 8" provides clear hurtsogood focus on a general point in intento-physical consciousness, greater distance, once the circuit is closed, gives me greater precision. Perhaps this focus is more specific than the basic moving contact and contract body consciousness loci outside of the head that are initially established. It seems now that such hand-independent loci establishment focuses similarly on healing energy complexes, while more-distant handtenna from further reaches in their tethered space may reach deeper and be more incisively focussed.

Instanding, two inner thigh muscles vibrate 1" outward as the rest of the body experiences imperceptible but palpable motion throughout.

Another day, a long slumped-seated *standing wave*, with two nodes above a grounding of the upper thighs at seat edge and in the area surrounding the atlas/occiput, is ridden full out to exhaustion as slight physical or intentional adjustments in the nodal points alter the wavelengths of the totally alternate state of feeling and dwelling only in the exhilarating restoring flows of body energy. Standing, these nodes are located and tuned simply by *intention* when the hands are connecting or after they are no longer needed.

When the *handtenna* are in closed circuit with internal foci of consciousness they are usually mirrored and the two points within move in their discovery in a matched way. Both *handtenna* or just the internal points can focus on one leg or all on a single point, however, when thus *intended*.

When the mirrored loci of *intention* move from inner leg around the mid-thighs while *instanding*, specific thigh muscles or groups tend to vibrate and visibly define themselves while the standing wave varies slightly.

Moving *hurtsogood* focus from top rim front to the sides of the pelvic girdle not only changes the standing wave nodal vibration quite a bit, but wobbles the spine undulation some and a point on the rim is found where each vibration from floor to occiput, though noded on the pelvic rim, dramatically clicks a thoracic vertebral energy cluster.

An interesting focus is around the perineum which seems the locus of leg/pelvic thrusting and rearing back. This directional balance vibrates between its states and creates one of the few omni-directional rotating thigh vibrations that don't self-destruct.

Once familiar, handtenna may activate or disengage on *intention*, but when this aerobic vibration session comes to a satisfactory release, I usually ground the hands against each other to put them to sleep.

Instanding and *waving* the second chakra muscles of standing and thrusting energy, here activated and regulated by the *protocol* and patterns of erect embodyment consciousness, are over-scene by a harmonic consciousness apparently anchored multi-dimensionally in the feet.

When you consider the number of energy contact nodes on the bottom of the feet and the number of ways from individually to multiply they might be combined while *instanding*, you get an idea of the full and partial harmonic spectrum of possible limp-muscled ligament and bone rattling that can be explored from that foot conSole.

I'm often aware of being in a harmonic beat with whatever music, and further examination seems to indicate that my currently in-play vibrating matrix of energy nodes chooses to modify its *waving* because harmonizing is at the core of *intentionality*. Besides, for example, there's again a large number of possible energies in a leg throughout and it may take a lifetime to get them back into the natal harmony unless you give them free rain (*water prana?*).

Today, after some aerobic thrusting-noded *waving* ending with almost full legs quite animatedly vibrating ahead of me from a chair, alternately or in tandem, I 'pressed down' not by grounding, but on the intentional image of the foot conSole and then varied that ungrounded out there *waving* in one or another or both legs by the 'pressure' I differentially 'applied'.

More and more the *intentional* image of where consciousness is *intended* to be directed supplants the need for a direct hand-to-body *transducing* of the coursing body energy. Imaging hard-to-access between-the-shoulder-blades energy out in front of my consciousness, for example, I work rooting and routing around in that general shoulder/spinal body province with handtenna 16" on either side of that image in front of me and interlocked to time-space. Then the hands swing around behind in a reach I can not normally accomplish, below about 20" away and focused upon that same area with the same *intentionality*.

Learning that the foot conSole is really a place in my consciousness accessible by *intention* suddenly opens and extends this nodal exercise program to an additional spectrum of fish-like *waving*, while lying on the back – a new approach to releasing this energy.

Lying, and raising my feet, I press upon the conSole and activate the stiffly-elevated legs into a number of fierce *waving* harmonies. Then, rotating the extended feet incrementally, different affects of rapid vibration are accessed, probably in the same octave.

Relaxing down the feet from their erection, the same *waving* could be played while lying body-limp, including focus on a single mid-arch point on the bottom of each conSole that, when *intention* overtook it, expanded to a center-penetrating light shaft and triggered full bodied *waves* (hence the fish image). Not just gentle *waves*, but end lifters and bottom thumpers. Harmonic flopping, extendable to aerobic extremes of post-orgasmic simplicity.

It is later discovered that focusing on pretty much the whole conSoles while lying limp on the stomach generates even greater flopping undulations rather hard to instigate voluntarily from this position with walking and standing and torso muscles. Stephen of my family showed me this, his butt arching a foot and a half in the air in an undulation that included his full length <u>independent of its resting support.</u>

I'm more and more becoming stateless. Stable states unintended and *intended* become very parallel realities and the protocol of switching between them has largely fallen away. I earlier thought that, once the this day in our time's *intended protocol* parameters had crossed my reality over, I had a little leeway to peer out, even report out, from that state altered from normal and I could probably return after being summoned by some urgency and could. It now seems that the *protocol* was a switching device that I have downloaded and can now execute simply *by intention*.

All of these 40 or so years of seeking inwards only minimally prepared me for the simplicity and elegance of *intentionally* switching consciousness. Thy will be done and all that. More, let's get out of here into the always parallel prana grounds to both experience, witness, and participate in our embodyment. I'm glad to say it - reality shifting is addicting. My consciously-chosen addictions have toyed with altered consciousness in the passed, but now a portal is open to *intentionally* rebirth my body for whatever else I had in mind with this encarnation.

That last sentence was a double heeder. Over 40 years ago people started to complain about my liberties and linguistic recklessness with living language. I speak German where if you know the spelling it is always pronounced the same and words that are syllably terminal can be combined literally and creatively at will to convey conceptual platforms with integrity. Like ideographs or American Sign Language. This idea has been very useful to me, as you have scene, to delineate knew concepts. I think of it as an inherent part of the *mirth* that is signature to these gnuer discoveries.

With a sense of ever increasing sureness concerning the ability to encompass in *intention* the more diverse lateral or rotating muscle energy chords that depart from ventral dorsal *waving*, when *intending standingwave* and with the hands perhaps moving intention, or with the ability of the rhythmic vibrational movement itself to focus consciousness specifically on one or a field of several energized moving especially vertebral muscle energy chordal nodes, I move *intention* to the ringed anchoring rim of connection between the thighs and the pelvis, starting at the sides, and discoverMoving the consciousness points incrementally around to the front or back when one, then several, rotational vibrations of discreet muscle band thongs stand strongly in the thighbed which is calmly *waving* in the dorsal ventral *(DV) protocol instanding*. This happens and next isolates inner-thigh thongs that feel anchored to the distracting second chakra energies; while outer thigh thongs tend to drag the whole thigh totally over to nodal *DV instanding*, but with a changed pitch to the *waving*.

When energy is *waving* the whole body, fully out-stretched overhead arms move in tandem high to the sides and to the rear in patterns usually no longer possible for me, even with pain that doesn't hurt so good. My left arm has long had a cramping with certain extensions that I feel mimics the right biceps stub that snapped when I returned from riding the bicycle for miles across the desert at Burning Man '99. When the right arm is *waving*, be it carrying the much accelerated upward and outward extension of the spine *instanding* and moving to activating the hands in any direction if they *intend* it, the perfect body of *intention* is where consciousness finds itself and where the harmonics of the energies of the earth course madly through every cell and hollow and where the body's template pattern is found and experienced to a *knowing*.

Friends, the auric body is where your reality is grounded.

Lying on the back opens and broadens *intention's* range of vibratory manifestation out from the predominant central energy flows. It accesses the hip nodal area's broad back fulcrum potential and thus triggered can move much further through the hip and leg energy body with concomitant *hurtsogood* (HSG?) guidance. The scapula/shoulder is also a broad nodeWork from which vibrations can be *intended* out. Both sacrum and hurt backside become *waving* nodal palettes for intuning vertebral linkage and energy transmission. With at least several tandem focuses of wave length influence, as with the foot consoles, these are harmonic conSoles playable and experienceable in locus-focus adjuvination.

On the back, with lower legs providing a vertical stand fulcrum and varying the pelvic upthrusting (hands clasped behind head) from the shoulders by pushing the feet conSoles broadly down – consciousness is abandoned to rhythm and wave length and wandering nodality up the snapping spine noticing and guided by affect. Your *intention* is running this complex Situation now. This 'stand' position can also be changed by bringing the tandem foot conSoles together twinning the affect of *intention* by grounding foot contact into itself into an aurobourous scissored by awakening knee energy flows, open-thigh-proffered auric genitals, and flexing a surrounding limb halo embracing the genital energies. I still can't quite have a full understanding of genital *intentions* and have colored my accessible image archives in many layers not flattened (Photoshop concept). Erotic images are so important that my bone sexuality insists that *my* bone be *that* bone and I'm not *intending* to go there. No bone will blossom here though, midst the halo around auric genital energy branching away from free energetic serpenspine confusion undulations.

Stroking with tandem *handtenna* an auric penis from 16", after rooting around the ventral pelvic floor and locating the auric balls for some intense *hurtsogood* exchange, a range of mostly other mostly penis images roams the magic theater let loose by *intention* soon to be interrupted by inhaling. So much happens on the exhale.

Even though I start from grounding for the *instanding*, grounding really has nothing to do with *waving*, but is a trigger to learn and to make it accessible to your *intentional* memory. It turns out grounding is a portable node in the larger rejuvenating action. After a while you can just simply image the grounding of your "grounded' console and crank 'er up.

It gets difficult for me when on and contacting rigid seating (like in a ME campground thunderstorm as I rite) not to vibrate my legs and let it go 'unintended' where it will as I try to write about it. Once triggered, that wave explorer has a mind-muscleloose of its own. More and more such blind wanderings result in complex semi-spastic omni vibrations that may interact their noded extensions from the rigid seat contacts to significant loft of lift off, neck rocking, or pounding butt or heels. Awareness of the detailed complexity of the frenzy is riveting. Sometimes the wave threatening spasticity becomes a sweeping and somehow already-learned-and-sensed tango. Rhythm is everything to supporting healing wave lengths and there can be multi-nodal rhythm in spasticity. Gets away from you though.

Total relaxing, so simple of skills, a forgotten way of being. When you can *intend* this state without short-circuiting the reality transition, the energy field is open for sure to its natal and still auric patternings. These one and the same templates abide with me and thee totally unique to each other but with great communality. Because of this relaxed reality interface between energies in tension and those at peaceful rest, those still-guiding template energies can be allowed to provide location and direction to moving consciousness and its circuitry. It's a little bit like the clapping game, the *hurtsogood* gives you directional readings. You must listen, Grasshopper.

Sitting on a relatively rigid seat seat, you touch down consciousness to the seat-full of generating butt nodes grounded when *in* this *situ*. Sensing three pairs of contact in rotation I note the different basal *waving* these three nodes moving 'down leg' from what must be the sitz-bone generate in mid ranges of vibration above basal *instanding waving*.

Sitting, the vibration of some major under-thigh muscle pack vibrating between sitz and knee rhythmically lifts me off at least an inch. This happens even when I think about it now. Focussing prana on the most 'down-leg' sitting contact on chair edge node elicits also counter-directional whole-leg-torso forward and back rocking-thrusting of a couple of inches knee movement. You find one of these set-ups and it is an easy ride for a while. Next, you raise the heels generating a new faster vibrational action adding the heels to the vibrational linkage and waving length.

Your new protocol world abandons virtually all of its external sensing and interacting and focuses on the energy that is streaming within it, and the exquisitely focused points of consciousness within its dynamism. This state has been previously glimpsed in the focus just before orgasm and in the viewpoint permeating all of your world during orgasm's extended tensionless overglow. After 10-15 minutes such focused absence from your usual self can actually be exhausting (a pranic breath term?), especially if your sojourn has been a lot of vibratory waving, however discrete.

Chaired on the back porch, midst shucking elderberries for this year's 300 wine bottles from my 35-year recipe, in and out of sun onto closed eyes, suddenly sitting in standing wave between buttocks and grounded feet with neck involvement promoting a rhythmic up and down speckled visual field around its golden radiating center, the rods and cones stimulated warmly by the sun. That field in the mind's eye, or aye, is the same one where *intention* places the images of body places it wants to focus on.

Gradually noticed is a warped matrix of blue sorta horizontal lines of lower case letters grouped in irregularly spaced pairs or triples that created no words or even syllables, i.e. had no relationship to conceptual communication. I remember g r t and n perhaps u – come to think of it possibly no other vowels. Now I'm not sure about t because I don't think there were any letter tops protruding above the ribbons. Letters vertically in the ribbons matched, I'm pretty sure. The turquoise-blue letters faded slightly as they radiated out. They were about this big, speaking for the six-lines-per-inch Verdana 10pt script you are reading. But how do you describe the size of a three-dimensional non object, and a lot of them moving fast? The ones I was looking at that half day like today are 8 lines to the inch size. And how do you evaluate sometimes blurry vision after more than a while, and you have not looked out the window to keep your focusing energy-complexes responsive, and you are already focusing from 2 ft to infinity (and beyond with the minds-eye) your 20/20 left far eye right brain closer than it likes to be, and the right 20/30 near eye left brain more comfortable from 9" to 24" is doing the more focused work, with the left eye fogging the resultant view of events put together when the two sides of the brain decide what thEye are seeing. I muse or amuse on the concept that size is really globally scene as the angle of view chosen. Since those partnered visionarys' view is an out-radiating as well as receptive pair of overlapping cones of consciousness, the mobial edges of which taper gradually into other wavelengths than visiospectral, size of any discovered objectivization in the mind's eye must vary.

I explored this extraordinary tapping-in to some spino-transmissional channel with the full body vibrations or disturbing some cerebral storage with residual information that needed release. This moving upward-only rolling sometimes stopping matrix, unlike the screen type I had just hunt-and-pecked the last three hours, which jerked occasionally downwards in bunches always in turquoise, which varied perhaps further from the orb and perhaps is influencing the spectrum of the popping dark void in its eccentric hieroglyphic radiation.

Never having been there or 'here' before, I compared the matrix of sometimes scrolling varying symbol ribbons with some strong multiplicities of images quickly accessible from those dozen or so ritual LSD and mushroom trips over the last 39 years (always with a porpoise), and can only indict that day's interaction with the monitor, where also would experience blurring maybe each time I have worked at length lately asking technology to give me an extended voice to awaken other people to their potentiality.

Next, I examined fear of snapping my head off or abrading a notch in my spinal chord for moving that which was retired from function against old will, while venturing on for five or so minutes playing and varying the nodes of contact for actual ground and for buttocks to suggest intended direction with everything coursing with expressed, harmonic, or just relaxed energy. The image superimposed on my innocent visual field was easily available to me still, next, as it had been during the fear examination terminated by simply asking the Self what is thy *intention*? And would it hurt you except for soGood? The matrix moved somewhat variably when I was still and when I was moving. In the rest of the body my energy burgeoned.

The shape and color was more important to rods than color, I would guess, so my rods must be seeking redress expressed to reverse the aggressive visual impact in the very ground of my intended void. The wraiths are gone now, we'll see if they reappear today after sending my 220 pg 5th and most important book for change off to Lulu yesterday and today spending five hours with garden in between at it.

One theory is that residual radiation from the screen in the visual receptors might express in the turquoise blue rod range, but I don't think that's it. I used my trifield meter to check magnetic output from the screen and found 1.2 milligauss on the screen and only .3 milligauss 16" away, about the same low radiation as from my computer 16'" away from my right knee. Three feet away from my recent 19" screen TV measures 4 milligauss, or 4 kiloVolts/meter. I can't measure actual radiation coming from radioactive components of a screen, only magnetic and electric fields, but from considerable research on radiation's affects described in the last chapter i don't think there's any danger from these screens as they are used and .3 milligauss is 300 volts/meter, when sustained 1,000 vpm can be said to harm.

So what's residual? All I can think of is the constant contrast of fixed size letter figures on ground might by stressing the light intensity receiving cones, along with the right eye left brain having to over-perform at keeping the dis-focussing left far-seer at bay in their mutual translation. Being a hunt-and-pecker, my eyes are also always focused during input time on the letters on the keys in continual passage. Another thought I have today is remembering the solar dappling of the eyelids as the zephyrs tousled the shading Rowen tree. Light protons come through lids. As well, the Ultra-Violet generates Vitamin D-25 which elicits a seratonin lift to the first cells it reaches and perhaps where it permeates to the retina, knowing that the cornea would transmit these wavelengths as glass on our face won't. This memory lingers on in my gallery.

I often hear my inner dialog asking How can you not think about something when that thing is not thinking? (We must have solved this younger, no?) Meditation is focusing your energies toward the exclusion of external and internal triggering and comfortably doing lurking-time. When your protocol gets you there it is to astound how thin the barrier between states is sprung with *intention*. The enthusiasm with which each state of full consciousness ever becoming more desired is approached facilitates our moving, whenever possibly in life, in meditation. More *in there*, yet also *out there*. (Oops, vibrating a bit as I write I almost just stumbled on a threshold of left-over *nontentions*.) (I can't figure that out either.) That's *in there* and *out there* too. More and more separating out my incessantly narrating and commenting-on-the-narration voices that seem to run in both *theres* of *being here*, has been teaching me, as always. I can use them (both speak German occasionally, often when perplexed) in both states to narrate out, as well, and to report visually without state degradation. Just as when being present one can lapse into another state I also have zum Beispiel (e.g.) a *creative* altered state, not yet factored in.

A voice Should I write about it comes in strongly. Some challenging voice says sarcastically Oh yeah. When it goes on they each comment on each other – not sure who's dictating the often apparently unrelated things Seth taught me to gather in my spare time. It used to be voices chattering Who can I share this experience with halfway through the teaching in order to show I'm learning how to justify my being. All our voices know now that we are able to see more than the beginnings of change in the makeup of our entire coursing energies.

I look out from my ever-undulating swing chair, with eyes autonomically keeping grasp on the 10% of the visual that the thalamus lets through, a constrained larval entity on an accelerated expansion beyond conventional mind washing depiction, and regularly pupate when in *intended* altered body states. The rhythm of the often complex movement connects me with the porch glider I slept on during teen summers when that moving/sleeping came to unconsciously launch me into Robert Monroe's trips out-of-body. It harks back too to still-influencing Jean Houston's conversion in her group therapy books and teachings, when she could no longer use psychedelics, to witches cradles – swinging chairs – and her use of monotonous repeating motion states to alter the states of most entities. The repetitively and tunable complex full or partial interacting body vibrations, when the rotation of the chair itself is vibrating with the nodal one or two paired points of body contact with it, remains sustainable generally only if ventral/dorsal, because that matches the chair's direction of swing. Side to side body waves sometimes harmonize with *instanding* waves creating a complex tango-like partial body or full gyrations until sustained monotony can be reached.

Genitals stay shrunk and get very blue when the pelvis is the nodal focus. My next project is to film a lot of these daily body sparkings. Today would have shown how much sweat was generated on an entity that normally doesn't and uses no soap in about 5 minutes of one thrusting *instanding* with a long focus in the neck slide and more than usual head participation in the wave. When a strong vibration is encountered to stay current with, nodes can be vibrated within it without, or perhaps only slightly, changing the frequency bent. With video I might be able to establish what the various full body frequencies are and examine their body harmonics. When I film it'll have to be full body and not because the *handtenna* aren't able to 'reach' through to matter in its intended location, with perhaps only a coursing psi connection. Also, since I have come to deal with the energies of my sexuality with its target location in my mind's eye, aye, somewhere in front of me, my full cover will have to be blown to see how the vibration often focused on cock or balls or buttocks or inner thigh affects those regions usually 'draped'. Besides, with video you get to see a totally relaxed jaw and facial muscles quite distorted except when moaning exultantly. What I am fascinated to see is the form and movement of the *handtenna* dance, as the body's full access to its three dimensional matrices performs without any conscious direction.

I am learning that the body operating under auric connection to its energies accesses the full articulation of its various vortexes of interrelated activity. When the hands are connecting the body's vibrational circuitry (they long since need no protocol to activate with *intention*), whether in psi contact with a physical body location or with its intended image wherever you place it, the hands are in perfect mirror sync unless intended otherwise (say, both working on the right leg). This synchronization is at quite another level than that possible under conscious volition.

3 pages for the next 7th edition expansion without having to change the Table of Contents each time

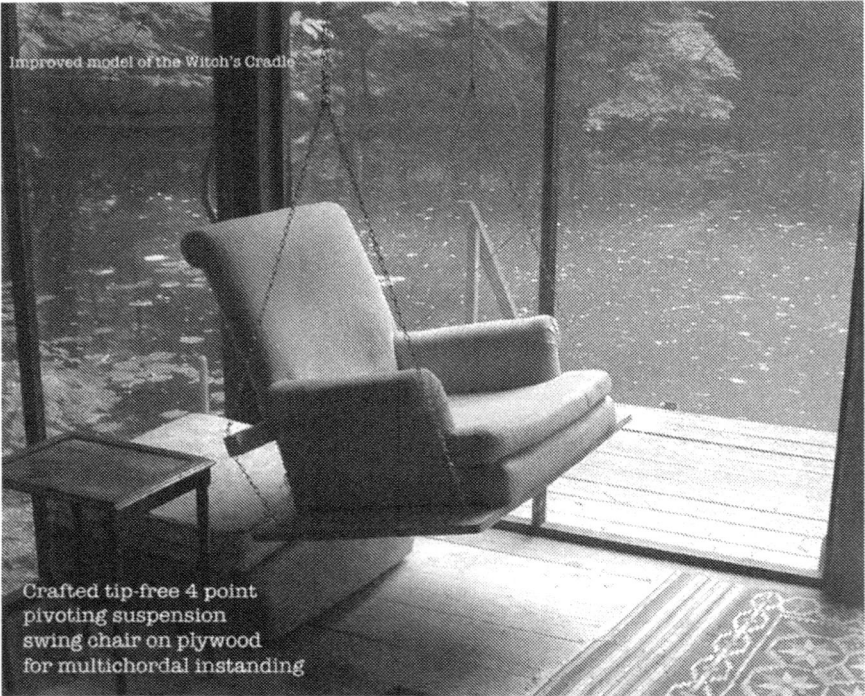

Improved model of the Witch's Cradle

Crafted tip-free 4 point
pivoting suspension
swing chair on plywood
for multichordal instanding

I keep collecting notes, but this is enough to give you an idea of the places your *intention* can lead you. Our embodiment is similar, but my entity's unique ontology, maturation, and 77-year mellowing provides its unique pattern of manifestation, and my healing path to adjuvenation and to reclaiming the energy flow of the natal body will be similar in mapping, but different in expression from yours.

For me, stretching the exhale to its limits and beyond is opening to the flow of palpable body energy that can be accessed by vibrational resonance, coupled with a protocol portal accessing hitherto unrealized properties activating the hands as transducers of energy to be listened to and followed. This much will work for you and your *intention* will take it where it then needs to go in order to heal thyself.

Energies of the Body

The body can be conceived of as being an orchestral manipulation of waves and pulses among biological oscillators with variable inherent sustainability, coherence, and harmony. The regulation of all this activity of living has our modified reptile and bird brains, shallow and deep, shimmering wavelengths and complex harmonies or disharmonies of vibrational expression, playable electronically on our EKG or EEG console along with energetic and emotional cranial to sacral primal tides, with even cells' communication with UV light transmission and reception along non-existent pathways, not to mention the influencing of considerable advanced cellular chemistry. Every time you pick off a piece of the body to examine, you wind up having to look at the whole thing as well as what's also around it.

It is the wave length synchrony, the harmonic relationship of the brain's agitation with the field phenomena like Schumann Waves that provide the battery driving life itself, which pumps the spine juice called Kundalini and facilitates suffusing every cell with ECK in stasis, the ecstasy for which living cells are programmed to yearn. Success in the balancing out of these converging vibrational energies comes with perfected **embedding**, which seems to describe the goal of bringing the vibration of living, earth influence of gravity, centering, reaching energy to others (compassion), and self-awareness, all into being self-referent through the Golden Mean PHI Ratios, thus enabling these vibrations to reenter themselves non-destructively – producing living harmony. Simply stated, a large number of the oscillating harmonics of our living, of our waking, walking, talking, and thinking being cannot exist co-constructively if the ratios between those diverse harmonics anchored to earth energy are not harmonics of a power series of the golden ratios of PHI. This mathematical ratio of 1 : 1.618, also called the Fibonacci Spiral, spins energy from one state to another by shifts in frequency ranges creating broad spectral coherence in EKG. The moment when the most number of harmonics can inhabit an oscillator like the EKG is when those harmonics fit recursively into the geometry of perfect PHI self-embedding (in Resonance with the Vibes).

The word PHYsics means literally the Science of the cycles of PHI. This is pure principle. Science means literally: "to love to know" or "to know to embed".

The body is the garden of the soul (<u>Angels in America</u>). It seems that, when we get inside the body and want to ask about its zillion pieces communicating with each other to create an intentional community in resonance with earth energy, after dealing with the amino acids and hormones of nerve communication like *norepinephrin, melatonin, cortisol,* and *serotonin* and lots of other chemical conversants which work specifically within nerve cells, **waves of visible light turn out to be our basic intercellular AOL**. Remember, there's some 1,300 nerve endings served by neurotransmitters in one square inch of skin, but 19.5 million cells on that square inch also yearning to work in tandem with the goals of the entity that brought them together. Other chapters have somewhat surveyed the place of ELF waves in harmonizing the overall brain and body functioning with earth energies and the deleterious effects higher human-made waves and magnetism are certainly having upon the species and its host planet. Einstein's Theory of Relativity concludes that light is in some ways more fundamental than either time or space. As we embrace, here, **light's full spectrum**, we include for consideration all of life as well as our inner light which radiates out into the world. We understand ourselves to be "light beings". As Goethe said, " The inner light will shine forth from within us, and then we shall need no other light". Light is the principle underlying all manifestation. **We, our bodies and our minds, are light**, said Georg Feuerstein.

Around 137 million photoreceptors in each eye transform light into electrical impulses for the brain. Light is a major factor in our health, and affects the mental, emotional, and spiritual bodies that are causing disease, allowing a client, when it is used therapeutically, to look at what is happening emotionally, mentally, and spiritually. How each of us responds to colored light is as unique as our fingerprint. In Europe, color therapy is considered to be a medical procedure.

When I have written of healing my near-sighting by restoring elan to the ciliary muscles by ultra-violet wavelength bathing, I was championing all muscles' and immune systems' full spectrum of sunlight needs, and their dependency upon specific wavelengths of that light which could be received through the eyes and the skin in the ambient light of shade. This approach is close to a large field of phototherapy or syntonics, which has evolved to stimulate the biochemistry of the brain through the visual system, by way of the retinal-hypothalamus brain connection. **Syntonics** treats a wide range of visual dysfunctions of eye movement, including learning disorders and the after-affects of stress and trauma. Treatment of Seasonal Affective Disorder with blue light is a syntonic type of therapy. Resetting the circadian clock is much involved here, with very specific wavelengths in the visible spectrum having very expectable effects.

Syntonic Optometry fans out to include all aspects of visual functioning, including academic achievement, athletic performance, and proficiency at work. Dr Harry Wohlfarth found lighting and wall colors even carpet colors, influenced school attendance, performance, and academic achievement. John Ott found lighting closely simulating sunlight's spectrum affected health, behavior, and performance in classrooms and offices. In 1985, psychiatry belatedly discovered light therapy as a treatment for SAD, and medicine on this continent is investigating light therapy for jet-lag, PMS, sleep disorders, and other circadian rhythm disorders. Dr Jacob Liberman's 1991 book Light: Medicine of the Future further amplified the role of light and color in health, proving improvement in visual skills, peripheral vision, memory, behavior, mood, general performance, and academic achievement.

James Lovelock demonstrated in 1989 that **cells themselves communicate with one another coherently by the exchange of photon quanta**, opening to science a wider field of visible-light wavelength understanding. Szent Gyorgyi, Herbert Froelich and Ilya Prigogine (Nobel laureates) and, in 1974, Fritz-Albert Popp, have shown that nucleated cells, by way of physical and vibratory configuration of their DNA, are capable of picking up, storing, and broadcasting information (order and negative entropy) about their environment. The biophoton theory, developed on the basis of these discoveries, says that **ultra-weak photon emissions of biological systems are weak electromagnetic waves in the optical range of the spectrum (light) emitted by living cells of plants, animals, and human beings which can be measured**. **This dynamic web of biophotonic light, constantly released and absorbed by the DNA, may serve as the organism's main communication network and as the principal regulator for all life processes**. The holographic biophoton field of brain and nervous system, perhaps the whole organism, may be the basis of memory and other aspects of consciousness (postulated by neurophysiologist Karl Pribram, and others). Since its base is in the properties of the *physical vacuum,* it may play a significant role in the non-physical realms of mind, psyche, and consciousness.

Scientific support is given to healing methods unconventional to Western medicine by the discovery and investigation of this biophoton emission. The meridians of "ch'i" energy, which Traditional Chinese Medicine considers to regulate our bodily functioning, may be related to node lines of the organism's biophoton field, as well as the "prana" of Indian Yoga. Popp discovered that the light is emitted from nucleated cells "bundled" and directional, like laser light. This speed of light can be seen as necessary for communication throughout the body **- the biochemical processes are subtly magnificent, but too slow for total body consciousness**. Biophoton light also leaves the body, noticeably from the eyes and the aura, networking living things into Rupert Sheldrake's morphogenetic fields.

The practice of acupuncture dates back 5,000 years in China. The Taoist philosophy holds that the interaction of two forces, Yin and Yang, creates a body energy that flows through 12 plus 2 meridians which, like electrical currents, connect to focal acupuncture juncture points. This system, separate from the nervous, circulating, and lymphatic systems, is one of directional flow, with turn-arounds in the extremities, generally moving from hand to head to feet to chest region and back to hand. These flows can be measured with Kirlian photography, which records bioelectrical and biophoton measurement, especially as they 'leak' from the hands and feet. Robert Becker concluded that the meridian system is "involved in the receipt of damage or injury stimuli which we perceive as pain, and in the control of various processes of repair, including regeneration. Its nature renders it susceptible to perturbation by electrical and magnetic fields and it is proposed that it furnishes the linkage mechanism between biological cycles and geomagnetic cycles." Acupuncture points have higher electrical conductivity and thus lower electrical resistance than other areas of the skin surface. Kirlian photography shows flares emanating more intensely from the points than from surrounding skin areas. At the moment that solar flares occur on the sun, there are changes in the electrical potential of the skin's acupuncture points.

David Icke's Newsletters @DavidIcke.com explores all aspects of energy. March 11,2007, in "Robots That Can Think", he wrote of the human computer:

The body's circuit board is the meridian system that forms the basis of the ancient healing art of acupuncture. Thousands of years ago the Chinese knew about the network of energy lines passing around and through the body that are now called meridians. Along these lines are many points, known as acupuncture points, where the flow of energy through the meridians can be regulated by using hair-like needles and other techniques. You can see in the image below how **the meridian system even *looks* like a circuit board**. This is a computer-enhanced version of an image produced at the Necker Hospital in Paris in a joint study with the Cytology Laboratory at the Military Hospital.

They injected a radioactive tracer into acupuncture points and then took the photograph with a gamma camera to see where it would go. It followed the pattern of the acupuncture meridian system. Not only does this confirm the existence of the meridian network, which 'modern medicine' has long dismissed and ridiculed, the study also established another crucial fact. They found that the slower the energy, or *chi* to the Chinese, passed through the meridians the less healthy was the person involved.

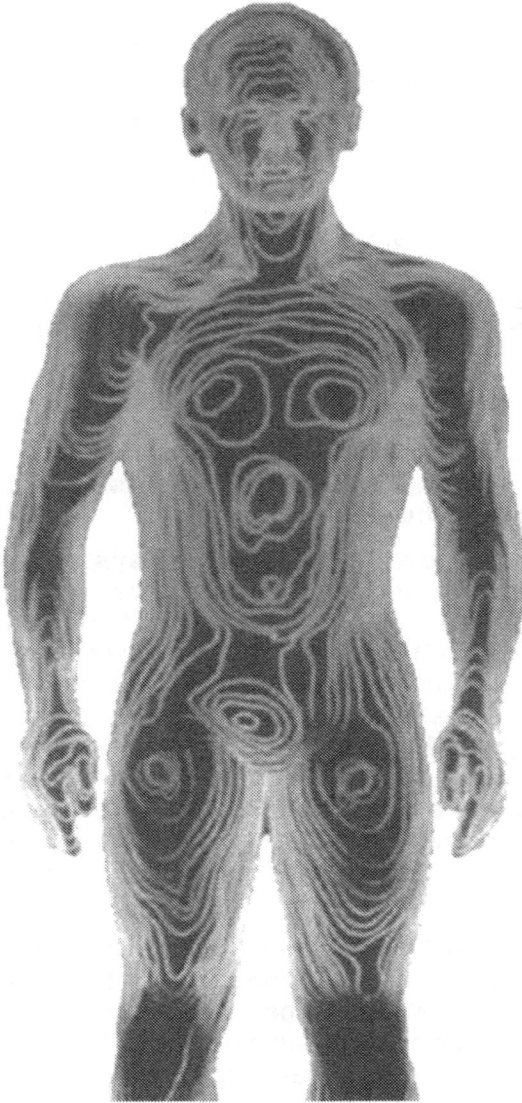

When the energy was flowing at optimum speed and balance the subject was in good health. How can this be? Because the energy, the *chi*, is *information* that includes details about a problem or imbalance and the instructions on how to respond. If people were taking too long to tell you that a problem exists and too long to pass your response to those at the scene what would happen? The problem would not get fixed and would probably worsen as a result. This is one reason why people who are ill are more open to other illnesses.

The *chi* also carries instructions that maintain balance and harmony and when this communication is affected so is the balance and harmony and the body becomes dis-*eased*. **The first thing you notice when a computer begins to malfunction is that it's slower than normal to respond to your instructions. Once that happens it can go on to become far worse unless action is taken to clear the system of whatever is slowing the communications traffic. So it is with the *chi* in the body circuit board.**

Those who have no understanding of how the body works, or even what it is, have long laughed at acupuncture and other 'alternative' methods of healing. Their ignorance cannot grasp how putting a needle in the foot or leg could cure a headache, for instance. This is because they associate the pain with the *location* of the pain when the body has to be seen as a whole.

The meridians form circuits around the body and a line that passes through the head also passes through the leg and foot. A blockage in those areas can cause disharmony elsewhere on the circuit and so restoring the flow at a point on the foot or leg can remove the pressure or other problem causing the headache. Computer technicians do something similar when they 'clean up' a computer to make the electrical circuits flow at optimum speed. These technicians are often referred to as 'computer *doctors*'. How very apt.

Because the body is a computer, albeit of fantastic sophistication, it can be programmed with 'software' and it is - all the time. **We inherit a hard drive from our parents with programmes already running and we download others through experience. The body is a biological computer in that it has the ability to think and feel emotion, both of which are electrochemical phenomena, and unless higher consciousness intervenes 'our' thoughts and emotions just follow the programmes.**

Control of humans is through control of the human computer and its thoughts, emotions and perceptions. This is why the understanding that we are infinite consciousness and not our bodies has been suppressed for thousands of years through religion and 'science'. Once we know who we really are we can open our computer minds to become truly conscious and override the software programmes we call perception and behaviour.

David Icke also says:

The Matrix trilogy and "Robots to be programmed with a code of morals so they won't attack humans" is not as far fetched as it may seem at first sight, not least because many of the foundations of the story are happening today. The other-dimensional entities manipulating our world or reality through a network of 'human' bloodlines - the 'Illuminati - are using us as an energy source by trawling low-vibrational emotional energy based on fear. This includes stress in all its forms and other expressions of fear like guilt, anger and vengence.

Society has been structured by these entities through their interbreeding 'human' bloodlines to induce maximum stress and fear and thus the energy they need to function. When people feel fear or other such emotions you can see the effect in their behaviour and feel the 'vibes' of the energy being generated, but **you can't actually see the energy because it is produced on frequencies beyond human sight. These manipulating entities operate in that frequency range and so when we produce fear and its low-vibrational offspring we are empowering those who seek to control us.**

We talk about creating robots when the world is already teeming with them. They're called humans - those humans who are not fully conscious and operate only at the five-sense or 'body' level of perception and reality. When we identify who we are with the body - I am Bill Jones, I am Ethel Smith - and forget that we are infinite consciousness we allow the body 'robot' to dictate our lives. And it is through the 'robot', the body computer, that the other-dimensional control is routed.

The body is an incredibly sophisticated computer, as I have shown in my last two books, *Tales from the Time Loop* and *Infinite Love is the Only Truth - Everything Else is Illusion*. The membrane of every human cell is a liquid crystal and, depending on who you ask, we have between 50 and 75 *trillion* of them. **Our cells are computer chips**. Bruce Lipton, a research scientist and former medical school professor, produced a detailed study of the cell membrane in his book, *Biology of Belief* (Mountain of Love/Elite Books, Santa Rosa, California, 2005). He concluded that **'the membrane is a liquid crystal semiconductor with gates and channels'. These 'gates and channels' open and close in response to electrical impulse to allow in the good stuff and**

defend against the toxic.

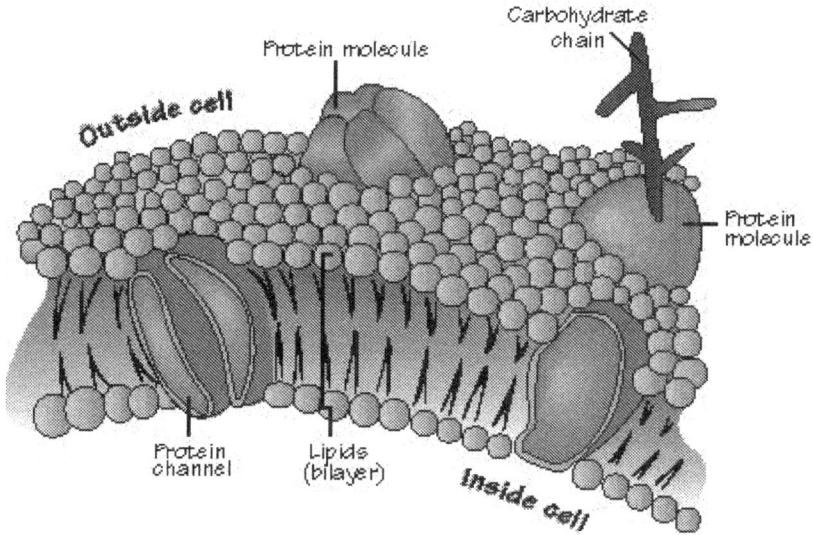

A human computer chip

Semiconductors are excellent conductors of electricity and can also be used as insulators. They are found in electrical devices like *computers*, digital audio players and cell phones and they are at the heart of microprocessor chips and transistors. Anything that is computerised or uses radio waves depends on semiconductors and here we have a semiconductor liquid crystal membrane on every cell. The principle component of semiconductors used in our electronics and chips is the silicon crystal, hence the term 'Silicon Valley' in California and the 'silicon economy'. Shortly after Lipton realised that **the cell membrane was a 'liquid crystal semiconductor with gates and channels'**, he picked up a book to see computer chips defined as ' ... a crystal semiconductor with gates and channels'. He writes:

'I spent several more intense seconds comparing and contrasting biomembranes with silicon semiconductors. I was momentarily stunned when I realised that the identical nature of their definitions was not a coincidence. The cell membrane was indeed a structural and functional equivalent ... of a silicon chip.'

The cells are, in part, the hard drive of the body computer with the crystalline DNA holding the genetic memory. The central processing unit or CPU is called the brain. A CPU is actually known as the 'brain of the computer' because, like the human brain, it reads, controls and processes all communications traffic.

The brain decides what to make of information, how to respond and where it should go. We should remember it is the brain that receives the information from the five senses and decides how to decode them. If you can manipulate and program the brain to read these messages in a different way you can get someone to eat an apple and yet taste a banana. Skilled hypnotists do this sort of thing in their stage shows. We don't feel pain at the location of a blow; we feel it when the information about the blow has reached the brain to be decoded into 'ouch!'.

So matter is a densification of light. There is a model of reality that I first ran across in Germany, which describes 9 dimensions beyond our three-dimensional manifestation, called "Lightbody". It was revealed by Tashira Tachi-ren, an entity channeled into this planet for a period of 12 years. 'Lightbody' says that the next, or fourth dimension, is not time, as we think of it, but is called the astral plane. It is "basically emotionally based" and the four lower dimensions together are "the dimensions where the game of separation is carried out". In this model, the planet and we are "in a state of ascension and currently vibrating at lower levels of this astral plane." (in a 'harmonic' state, perhaps?) "As part of the ascension process, all of the dimensions will be rolled up into the higher dimensions and will cease to exist". Here, too, is a possibility for 2012, if our evolution continues to accelerate.

The fourth, astral, Lightbody level holds the majority of your karmic patterning within the etheric body. It "also works to keep your DNA functioning at limited survival-based levels by inhibiting the amount of light your body can absorb". The fifth dimension of Lightbody is completely spiritually oriented, while the sixth "holds the templates for the DNA patterns of all types of species' creation, including humankind. It is also where the Light languages are stored and it is made up mostly of color and tone. It is the dimension where consciousness creates through thought [Ramtha's Void?] and one of the places where you work during [lucid?] sleep. In the fifth dimension of Lightbody is where biophotons and Eastern chakras come together. "The fifth dimensional etheric blueprint of Lightbody is made up of an axiotonal meridian system, an axial circulatory system, and spin points through which these systems and structures are connected." These axiotonal lines "exist independently of any physical body or biological forms" and are "equivalent of acupuncture meridians that can connect with the Oversoul and resonant star systems." The axiotonal lines are made of Light and Sound, connect meridians, and have "spin points" which are "small spherical vortexes of electromagnetic energy that feel like they are on the skin surface". There are also **spin points in every cell of the body which "emit sound and light frequencies which spin the atoms of the molecules in the cell at a faster rate. Through the increased molecular spin, light fibers are created which set up a grid for cellular regeneration."** Atomic spin, especially of hydrogen atoms, is a force akin to magnetism that science is currently trying to somehow harvest for profit to utilize for computer chips.

Cells metabolize light, shuttling energy back and forth between *adenosine di-phosphate* (ADP)' "an energy storing compound", and *adenosine tri-phosphate* (ATP), with the ATP molecules acting as an **antenna/prism** putting usable color frequencies back into the DNA strands. The Lightbody model includes chakras and other planes of consciousness which will not be covered here. What I think the model gives good conceptualization to, and helps us to understand, is the ancient Chinese ideas about the life force "ch'i", which plays itself out in meridians and acupressure points, with the chakras lurking in the background. When talking about body energies, we all occasionally allude to chakras. I am going to give as short a description of them as I can, and if you don't want details, skip over this.

Biophotons (and Wilhelm Reich's derided "bions") are things of the visible color frequencies. Ramtha defines "frequency" as "vibrating speeds that characterize a wave of energy, used to describe the vibrating rate of particles and waves *of a particular plane of existence*." I might say *of a particular plane of consciousness.* Energy "is the counterpart of consciousness. All consciousness carries with it a dynamic energy impact, radiation, or natural expression of itself. Likewise, all forms of energy carry with it (sic) a consciousness that defines it." The chakras each describe psychological views of the world, in order of ascension from the material to the spiritual levels. I am going to describe the Chinese system, with its relationship to color and body energies, and then return to Ramtha's somewhat different explanation.

Chakras are antennae. A chakra is a "wheel" or focus of energy in the body represented in the forms of plexuses and endocrine glands. Their perceived function is to gather energy from the cosmos, process it, use it, and even release it back. Each chakra "antenna", or level of consciousness, supplements a particular organ in its area or endocrine gland with **prana energy**, maintaining a healthy balance between the individual's subtle bodies (or **intention**) and the physical body as well as reaching into the whole bio-energic system. Chakras are independent and interconnected centers which influence each other. A dysfunctional chakra leads to energic imbalances, physical illnesses, and emotional blocks in the energy system. The human body has 7 in-body chakras and, if you believe this or perhaps can experience this model, one 6" below you in the ground, and one 12" above your head. They all have, as well as glands, organs, and body parts to tune, colors of the electromagnetic spectrum associated with them (light waves, biophotons) as well as (in various systems) elements, vowel sounds, stones, and essential oils. And, of course, positive and negative metaphysical qualities and influences, largely under-described here. I am interested in the light and color part.

Red has the lowest vibrational rate in the visible spectrum, thus it affects the most dense material matter in our organisms. Deep red/infra-red is the color for the chakra 6" under you in the direction of earth's core, while the first *root/base chakra* at the base of the spine (adrenal glands, bladder, genitals, spine) is red and is involved with instinct and self-preservation. It is associated with the earth. The orange-related *navel chakra* (reproduction, uro-genital system, kidneys, gonads, legs) is concerned with sexuality, pleasure, self-esteem, relationships, desire. Above the navel, below the chest, the *solar plexus* is associated with fire and the color yellow (digestion, solar plexus, nervous system, muscles). It energizes the nervous system, metabolism, digestion, emotions, focussing on personal power, self-control, warmth, and humor. Associated with the *heart chakra* is the color green, along with the element air. Controlling heart, thymus gland, circulatory system, arms, hands, lungs, it anchors the life force from the Higher Self and energizes the physical body and blood in its circulation. Divine/unconditional love, forgiveness, compassion, and peace are its blessing. The *throat chakra's* color is blue and the associated element is ether (the 'physical vacuum'?). The organs of the mouth and throat and upper lungs are its province, and the functions of communication. True communication, peace, truth, knowledge, wisdom, loyalty, responsibility are among its qualities. The *brow chakra, or third eye*, associates with indigo and *full-spectrum white light itself*. **Overseeing the pituitary**, left eye, nose, eyes, spine it vitalizes the cerebellum, central nervous system, and vision. Its metaphysical qualities are soul realization, intuition, insight, imagination, perception beyond duality, inspiration, and spiritual awakening, among other wonderful attributes. The element of the violet *crown chakra* protruding from the top of the head is, of course, thought and will. It is involved with the **pineal gland,** cerebral cortex, central nervous system, right eye. It vitalizes the upper brain and works toward the unification of the Higher Self with the personality. Oneness with the infinite, divine wisdom, selfless service, perception beyond time and space, continuity of consciousness, connection to inner guidance are among its attributes.

A functional summary of this traditional model is as follows – the source of our primal hungers and survival drives is in the first chakra situated in the genital region, forming our basic attachment to the material world. The main connection locus between the emotional and physical body and the primary connection to sexuality, anxiety, and pleasure is in the second or "gut" chakra. Connection between the intellect and reason, and the body resides in the third chakra, where the structuring, logical mental self is joined with the physical. Adolescence sees these three chakras open and functional, bringing essential bio-energy to the material, physiological, emotional, and mental aspects of our being - our essential inheritance. Higher self-knowledge and self-realization lies in the development of the next four chakras and an awakening awareness to the Higher-self, beyond the ego. The center of love and caring is in the heart chakra, which moves us beyond personal feelings. Motivated by desire or anger to a higher altruistic sense of compassion for others. Opening the throat chakra brings in divine will and higher authority and responsibility for one's actions and represents the capacity to lead others, to find your own voice, and to speak truth. The third-eye chakra opens to creative spiritual vision and leads to opening the crown chakra, the goal of yoga, or union with God.

Chakras have become much more real to me after knowing my intention is simultaneously strong enough to embrace them **in aura energy form** wherever I intend them and to feel their stirrings deep within my body. I elucidate my beginning experiences with learning to feel auras in the chapter on **psi Energy**. Pranic breathing is part of the Protocol.

As a speaking ascended master, **Ramtha's description of the planes of existence is somewhat different from Lightbody and the Chinese chakras.** The first three planes or "seals" are connected to our essential inheritance concerning the physical, emotional, and intellectual energies. In the second plane and seal, the infra-red frequency band is associated with pain and suffering. Magnetism is included here, too. This second plane is the negative polarity of the third plane of visible light frequency. **The third plane of consciousness with its seal dwells entirely in the visible light spectrum, between the red of suffering and pain and the ultra-violet destroyer of the old and creation of the new.** The fourth plane is "not yet split into positive and negative charge" (i.e. magnetically inclined). [As an aside – the art nouveauists and stained glass designers, as I often express, have had great difficulty capturing the iridescence of the ultra-violet. To me, it is a blending of both ends of the spectrum, a harmonic of red and blue that creates what Tibetans call "royal purple", also called 'blue' by Ramtha. Ramtha calls this fourth plane the Blue Plane and says that when it is lowered down to this solar plexus third plane of conscious awareness and the visible light frequency band, it splits into positive and negative polarity. "It is at this point that the soul splits in two, giving origin to the phenomenon of soulmates" (not defined). The fifth plane of *super consciousness*, associated with the x-ray frequency and the thyroid gland, relates with speaking and living truth without dualism. The sixth plane is the realm of *hyper consciousness* and associated with the pineal gland (third eye – melatonin regulator) and the gamma ray frequency band. It includes the "awareness of being one with the whole life experience. The brain is opened and true consciousness and energy is activated." The consciousness of the seventh plane, of an ascended master, is the Infinite Unknown frequency band. To understand all this, Ramtha recommends that "Truth is not mere data or information. **Truth is the full realization of a concept or paradigm of thought into experience and personal wisdom.**"

The symbolic writings of the oriental and occidental evolution systems and mysteries assure that a properly prepared spiritual aspirant can reach and attain up to three levels of consciousness, while still retaining an earth-bound existence when the physical and spiritual body undergoes spiritual transformative evolution with quantum energy products. Lymphatic, endocrinal, and etheric systems are involved, with the five spiritual chakras having physical counterparts in the spinal nervous plexus: coccygeal, sacral, lumbar, brachial, and cervical.

The five different chakras are able to be energized and opened along the spinal column of the 33 (degrees) levels up the spinal cord to the brain, with 20 nerves of the 33 spinal vertebra distributed one coccgeal, six sacral, four troublesome lumbar, five brachial, and four cervical. As the energy rises up the spinal cord vertebra by vertebra, each spinal nerve must be energized and opened up, each progressive spinal nerve and plexus energy attainment adds to the continued energy superconductivity of the spiritual aspirant's energy, with the full energization of each nerve-chakral entity harmonizing the multiple nerve frequencies together like notes, tones, and harmonic chords on an instrument. Each nerve has its own frequencies and the plexus has overtones, undertones and a harmonious chord.

The body develops a clearer rendition in whatever system - the spiritual body becoming alive with quantum energy, frequency, and corresponding sound - also becoming frequency color activated. Each frequency with its own undertones, harmonics, and overtone colors across the 33 spinal vertebra degrees of the body. The body becomes more conscious of itself, its interaction and communication with the extended world of materiality and living entities, and the activated lower endocrine organs produce physical hormones and spiritual hormones or psychic powers as a byproduct.

The second level of spiritual en-lighten-ment involves the pituitary and pineal glands maintained by 12 pairs of cranial nerves - olfactory, optic, oculomotor, trochlear, trigeminal, abducent, facial, vestibulocochlear, glossopharyngeal, vagus accessory, and hypoglossal. Full activation of the **pituitary** endocrine gland activates a multiplex of physical and spiritual hormones and a radiating aura in four directions from the frontal, temporal, and occiputal lobes, realizes the feminine energies of the body and consciousness and the first plane of cosmic consciousness. Full activation of the **pineal** endocrine gland manifests a radiant glowing golden blue white aura above the head - quadrant rays of royal divine electric blue-violet - and realizes the masculine energies of the body and consciousness - the second plane of cosmic consciousness. Marrying the masculine and the feminine to open a higher chakra and consciousness is stated to be the third plane of God consciousness.

These models, offering visible light's integral involvement with health processes, are largely considered to be fantasy and hoax by this nation's medical establishment. As it was with the Smithsonian, where a nation's responsibility for truth concerning ancient America was quite successfully subverted over a hundred-years ago by John Wesley Powell, the pernicious legacy of Morris Fishbein 'MD' (1889-1976), who is synonymous with the American Medical Association (the AMA has now become a more minor player among the **Four Horsemen of the For-Profit Apothecary**) has kept simple and accessible light therapy derided and suppressed. As new aquisitional and inquisatorial institutions became empowered and entrenched, the robber barons of the nineteenth century had discovered the profit value in technology and proceeded to exercise the same piratical control over intellectual property as they previously had over the short-lived age of enlightenment. Before 1913, the barons weren't yet enough organized to counterweigh the innovations of Alexander Graham Bell, George Westinghouse, and Nikola Tesla (namesake of my grandson Nikolai). **Morris Fishbein became Assistant Editor of <u>the Journal</u> for the**

recently formed American Medical Association in 1913 and Editor in 1924. His villanous legacy is of *ideocide*, and his suppression of health treatments with higher proven success than high-tech cut-burn-and-poison has proven an enduring genocide against all humanity. In the area of colored light therapies, Fishbein's persecution of Colonial Dinshah Ghadiali MD, DC, PhD, L.L.D. from 1924 to 1958, attempting to eradicate **Spectro Chrome Therapy (SCT)** from both practice and print, rivaled the FDA persecution of Wilhelm Reich (who died in prison in 1957 shortly before he was to become eligible for parole). Dinshah's low-tech accessibility and therapeutic efficacy, like many ideas of those three preceding him, provided an irresistible target for Fishbein and the healing-for-money establishment. Dinshah faced tribunals eight times. The first time was a victory for him, as only that time was medical evidence heard. He won the second trial trying to deport him because he was a Parsee "and a white man". The rest of the tribunals over the years he lost, as his lab was burned and all his equipment and all remaining records destroyed, he was forbidden to heal, and he spent 18 months of a five-year sentence in prison.

The fact that, for over half a century, medicine has **routinely** used (George) Westinghouse spectrally re-balanced blue wave-length enhanced maternity bulbs to treat neonatal bilirubin imbalance (jaundice), and that for as long, commercial breeders of chickens, chinchillas, and fish have been using John Ott's monochromatic reformulation work to manipulate fertility, gender, and behavior of animals that live in mal-illumined environments even as humans, is ignored by the medical establishment that bizarrely 'cares' for its cut/burned and poisoned patients under filtered 'cool-white' fluorescent hospital light rays and only allows FDA-determined minimum daily nutritive requirements. You want to change that, you have to call illumination '*only* cheerful', the co-enzyme pills '*only* food'. Those who chose to believe anything else without doubly blindfolded tests run by a for-profit manufacturer of wave length devices or nutrients, will be liable for suits involving civil, criminal, and professional responsibilities (particularly monetary liabilities).

Dinshah simply used *attuned coloured waves*, from any projected light source except fluorescent plus 12 coloured filters, and laboriously determined and charted his body *tonation* application formulas. The destroyed records would have been the significant heritage of his life-long work, recording, like Peter Mandel below, his thousands of clients and their *nitric oxide* realities. The very ease with which the proper *tonation* could be determined as sunlight with all its nutritive wavelenghts was absorbed by clients and could be applied by laypersons at home, constituted the true threat to the medical establishment. 1998 Nobel Prize winner R F Furchgott (*auf Deutsch* = 'Fear god"??) demonstrated the ability of light or photo energy to influence the localized production or release of *nitric oxide* and the stimulation of vasodilation through *nitric* oxide's effect on enzyme activity. This is the same province in which Viagra is working, and gay men have for decades been using *nitric oxide* (developed as a heart medicine) for their vasodilation needs well before Viagra (it's all acceptable now). Since the half-life of the *nitric oxide* which is released under the area and influence of illumination is very local (2 to 3 seconds), it prevents the effect of increased *nitric oxide* from being manifest into other portions of the body. 'FearGod' said that absorption is best achieved when light is 1) directed perpendicular to the skin, and 2) placed in direct contact with the skin. Moreover, photo energy emitted from a source that produces a homo-geneous wavelength is often more effective therapeutically than light composed of several wavelengths (for example white light).

A proprietary **Anodyne Therapy System** that delivers near-infrared (890 nanometers) photo energy from 60 super luminous diodes which are mounted on flexible pads that can be placed in direct skin contact, increases the localized microcirculation (which includes *nitric oxide*) by as much as 3200% after just 30 minutes, supplies 10 times more vasodilation (tumescence) than that which is achieved with warmth alone. The potential net effects of skin contact spectral illumination in relation to *nitric oxide* are, again, those of better blood flow, acute delivery of growth factors and white blood cells, fibroblastic differentiation and proliferation, angiogenesis, reduced edema, and the mediation of pain. Since they invented nitrous as an anesthesia almost a hundred years ago (I didn't check this) medicine has definitely kept its eye on 'Poppers'.

My daughter Meg was engaged in a series of phototherapy sessions involving 'colorpuncture'**, a**

systematic method of using colored lights applied to acupuncture points in order to facilitate the healthy exchange of information between the energies of the body and the mind. This language of light is one of Europe's most popular alternative healing techniques, originated 25 years ago by German scientist and naturopath Peter Mandel. **It has Dinshah P Ghadiala roots. With scientists now actually confirming light as the medium of intra-cellular communication of our bodies upon which our entire metabolism is dependent, colorpuncture, or esogetics, focuses coherent pure color frequencies using quartz glass pens, on acupuncture and other skin points**. Meridians actually light deep into the body, stimulating intra-cellular communication which supports healing.

For analysis in a therapy session, black and white Kirlian photographs of the energy emitted from the terminal points of the acupuncture meridians in the hands and feet are analyzed to point the practitioner towards the root cause of the imbalance in the bodymind. Follow-up light portraits after each treatment provide immediate feedback. The photo analysis, **based on analysis of some 800,000 photographs** over 20 years, often shows developing or pre-symptomatic stages of an energy imbalance, indicating preventative therapy directions.

Mandel's holistic paradigm for healing is a "merger of the esoteric wisdom of life with the energetic principles of life's process". Illness and pain are seen as segments where individuals may be blocked in their ability to manifest their potential or may have become distracted from their life path. Colorpuncture focuses extensively on expanding consciousness - bringing patients back in touch with who they really are and why they really are here. Working with pure light wavelengths, "esogetics is intended to help remove existing blockages and disorders, so one can travel one's life path freely and light heartedly"(sic).

Bhagwan Rajneesh (Osho) whose Active Meditations we did in the 70s, and who died in 1990, said his message "is not doctrine, not a philosophy. It is a certain alchemy, a science of transformation". Mandel was invited in 1989 to Osho International Commune back in Pune, India, to teach his method to a body of therapists doing research into the effects of color on the mind and meditation. Colorpuncture and Rajneesh''s Active Meditations seemed to complement each other well.

Dr Julian Whitaker's April 2004 Health Newsletter reports that his clinic has been using light just beyond the edge of the visible spectrum to treat diabetes complications and any "itis" of pain -- arthritis, tendonitis, plantar fasciitis, bursitis, fibromyalgia, carpal tunnel syndrome, strains, sprains and wounds. He has been using the FDA-approved *Anodyne Therapy* described above. As cells pass beneath the light unit, they absorb photons of energy, causing them to release *nitric oxide*, stimulating vasodilation and promoting better blood flow via stimulation of the enzyme *Guanylate cyclase* (GC) and facilitating acute delivery of growth factors and white blood cells, fibroblastic differentiation and proliferation, angiogenesis, reduced edema, and mediation of pain. Blue wavelengths supplied by similar pads to the surface blood vessels behind the knee cap are being used to alter the circadian clock in treating Seasonal Adjustment Syndrome. There are even light-based hair removal systems using a light source that produces non-coherent broad band pulsed light. The emitted wavelengths in this Swedish system range from 600 to 920 nanometers, with a special peak at 700 nanometers, which is the upper edge extension into the invisible infrared that is beyond the visible spectrum. That means that half of this wavelength energy working to eliminate those hair follicles is beyond the visible infra-red spectrum, and that half of the energy it is visible.

Meanwhile, in other frequencies, Peter Mandel has developed tools to regulate ELF brain waves as a way to support the body's healing processes, along with tiny crystals that adhere to acupoints after treatment to continue harmonizing these points.

In the realms of higher frequencies, sound, there are also therapeutic approaches. **Sonopuncture** is a practice in which high frequency sound is directed into acupoints. Sound waves have a well-demonstrated ability to rearrange particle sub-stances into complex geometric designs that support their arrangement totally in defiance of gravity fields (Cymatics). Sound is also used in bio-energetic healing. Research shows cancer cells unable to support the progressive accumulation of vibratory frequencies. Many different vibrating bodies are used. Tibetan brass bowls are awesome, but not as formidable even as a current therapy using very large bowl bells of the same shape fabricated from crystal. The re-balancing of potentials along the meridians is noted, with the effects being both physical, psychic, and holistic. Many therapies in the sound wavelength area (chanting) encourage involvement of the larynx as a creative organ with great balancing potential.

Sound is now used more and more **for bone healing**. 800 KHz is widely used through piezoelectric transducers generating ultrasound. Pulse frequency and total operating time in the use of electromagnetic stimulation of bone growth - osteogenesis - is postulated more significant for osteogenesis than pulse width or peak output. Electromagnetic devices producing direct, pulsed, or alternating currents usually have cathodes embracing a bone juncture or adjacent components. Also electromagnetic coils not in contact with the body are used, wherein a positive current appears to follow a circulating (eddy) current pattern in a fracture.

The optimal frequency for bone stimulation is 50 Hz. The dominant and fundamental frequency for three species of cat's purrs is exactly 25 to 50Hz - the best frequencies for bone growth and healing. The band frequency of cats extends up to 140 Hz, with all members of the cat species except cheetas having a strong or dominant harmonic at 50 Hz. The harmonics of three cat species falls exactly on or within 2 points of 120 Hz, a frequency which has been found to repair tendons. **Cats will purr when they are injured or in pain as well as when they are content**. Cats simply don't get chronic pulmonary disease, muscle and tendon injuries, bone disease, and a lot of other things that dogs get. In the Journal of the American Veterinary Association, Dr Gordon Robinson documented 132 cases of cats plummeting an average of 5.5 stories from high-rise buildings - some of them suffering severe injuries. 90% of these cats survived, with most cats that fell from seven or more stories managing to live. The record for survival from heights is 45 stories. The cat's purr is totally unlike any other animal's vocalization, yet the sounds of cats from 3 continents match exactly, in both amplitude and frequency. You may have noticed that when you are not feeling well your cat will often come up to the part of your body that's aching and start to knead you with their paws, purr, and get that meditative look in their eyes. They could be trying to help.

Scientists have discovered an amazing fact about the sounds of the ebb and flow of ocean tides, people's voices, dolphin cries, and bird and cricket chirps. They sound the same! When researchers slow down voice recordings of people, they discover the people's voices sound like the ebb and flow of ocean tides. Then when researchers speed up the recordings, people's voices sound like dolphin cries. Speeded up more, like bird chirps. Even more? Like crickets. And guess what crickets chirps sound like slowed down? Yep. First like birds. Then dolphins. Then people.

But wait! There's more. While examining recordings of spacecrafts Voyager I and II at the California Institute for Human Science, scientists discover the same sounds! NASA recordings from outer space sound remarkably like ocean sounds, choirs of voices singing, dolphins, birds and crickets. Additionally, sounds produced by the rings of Uranus are virtually identical to those produced by Tibetan bowls. Researchers believe that this similarity is no coincidence. Scientific medical studies are discovering that the sound vibrations of dolphins, Tibetan bowls, and choirs have a profound healing effect. Could this be the collective unconscious that Carl Jung refers to? A living collective library that contains all the knowledge of the Universe? Stay tuned!

-Center for Neuroacoustic Research and The California

I believe that **the chakras are nodes of the meta-meridians of the species-mind**. In contrast to all this, yet perhaps some confirmation of "all the atoms emitting light inside wavehood", here is a long quotation from Jack Keroac's <u>The Scripture of the Golden Eternity</u> that I am sure will help confuse you:

"All things and all truth laws are no-things ... in three ways, which is the same way: *as things of time* they don't exist and never came, because they are already gone and there's no time. *As things of space* they don't exist because there is no furthest atom than can be found or weighed or grasped, it is emptyness through and through, matter and empty space too. *As things of mind* they don't exist, because the mind that conceives and makes them out does so by seeing, hearing, touching, smelling, tasting and mentally-noticing and without this mind they would not be seen or heard or felt or smelled or tasted or mentally-noticed. They are discriminated from that which they're not necessarily by imagining judgements of the mind, they are actually dependent on the mind that makes them out, by themselves they are no-things, they are really mental, seen only of the mind, they are really empty visions of the mind, heaven is a vision, everything is a vision.

There's nothing to life but just the living of it."

Light is a local and distant communication system. On the more extended organic body level, one of the most significant harmonics of the expression of All-That-Is to be balanced enters from the deep resonating sound board in the curve formed by the cranium-compressed gate for **circulating cerebro-spinal fluid** on the top of the spine and the basal sacrum, a harmonic mirroring its flexion and extension and creating a pulse throughout the rest of the body; a sacro-cranial pump sucking UltraViolet out of gathered sex juices and pumping them 'thru the gates of the occiput' into the next harmonic in the coherent superconductive ecstatic process to super-nourish the high brain. **This pulse represents a third member in the musical chord of the breath and the heart-beat in the body.** It is the coiling serpent of kundalini. The spine juice long waves may exist "wave within wave", which is most sustainable – it is the musical key-signature to Cranio-Sacral tuning.

The body's **Cranio-Sacral System** is comprised of membranes and cerebrospinal fluid which form the fluid-filled sac around the core of the nervous system – surrounding, nourishing, and protecting the brain and spinal cord. With a total volume between brain and spine of 150 ml, a daily production of 500 ml replaces the fluid approximately every eight hours. It has a rhythm that can be felt throughout the body. Cranio-Sacral Rhythm is a very subtle rhythmical movement which is transmitted via the muscular, nervous, and fascial systems and the pulse can be felt (by Sensitives) anywhere on the body. Connective facia tissue is continuous from the top of the head to the bottoms of the feet. It is layered with pockets between layers containing the structures within the body such as organs, muscles, bones, etc. Normally, fascia is free to glide a millimeter or so and maintains a fairly elastic property.

John D Upledger describes "a triad of compression", completing a hydrodynamic membraneous circuit of the brain and spinal cord. The first compression or gate is at the lumbo-sacral L5 S1, the second is at the atlas axis C1 and C2, and the third is at the spheno-basilar junction, where the sphenoid and occiput join at the base of the skull. Upledger hypothesizes that the pulse of the circuit is created by the production of cerebral spinal fluid in the sinus ventricles of the brain. The ebb and flow of this cerebral spinal fluid creates a flexion and extension of the cranium and sacrum, creating a (joyful?) radiation of this pulse throughout the

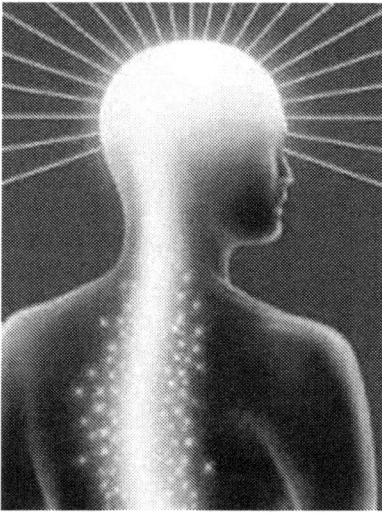

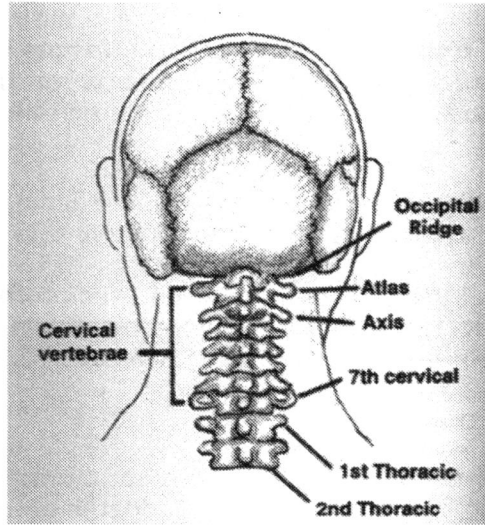

rest of the body. In order for these two ends of the triad to couple and link their movements in symmetry and harmony they must be mobile and free, If the cranium is not supported in free and resonant alignment with the spine, restrictions in the muscles, the connective tissues, and the over all energy of the body result. Synovial fluid movement depends on either the active or passive motion of joints. Restricted fluid movement leads to increased volume and fluid pressure, which can cause heightened tension, pain, and decreased range of motion.

Manipulative alternative medicine and rehabilitation therapies seek, at the tissue level, to restore optimal anatomic relationships, break down contractures or adhesions following long or short term tissue damage, and to improve fluid dynamics through the vascular and lymphatic circulatory systems. Different therapeutic approaches utilize a range of interventions from sustained forceful massage pressure across restrictive fascial bands to low or no-pressure stroking manipulative techniques connecting with the course of venous or lymphatic drainage to change fluid flow between and within tissue compartments. **One third of the 60% total body weight of water is extra-cellular, and the remaining two thirds is intra-cellular. Blood, lymph, and synovial fluid dynamics are affected by manipulation.** Fluid flow through the tissue interstitium is determined by hydrostatic, osmotic, and colloidal pressure gradients and protein concentration. **Application of oscillating compressive forces increases the rate of fluid interchange within and between intra and extra-cellular fluid compartments, which are always seeking connection.**

Human tolerances to whole body sinusoidal vibrations are listed for head pain at a large range of 13 to 30 Hz, with impaired speech in the lower half of that range, 13 to 20 Hz, and jaw pain (I can feel the throbbing of an infected tooth) a lower 6 to 8 Hz beat. Chest pain 5 to 7 Hz; abdominal pain 4.5 to 10 Hz; Lombotacral pain 8 to 12 Hz; urge to defecate 10.5 to 16 Hz; urge to urinate 10 to 18 Hz.

Some aspects of the urge to urinate are that, although the capacity of the urinary bladder is around 750 ml (about the size of a bottle of wine!), the stretch receptors start to respond when the volume reaches somewhere between 200 and 400 ml. Sensory neurons and sinusoidal vibrations send a message to the brain facilitating conscious desire to urinate, while from the sacral region of the spinal cord a reflex action of bladder contraction and internal sphincter relaction begins, with the external urethral sphincter awaiting conscious relaction.

Franklin Sills describes **cranial rhythmic impulse**, the fluid tide and cranio-sacral tissue motion and mobility, with a potential tide of 8 to 14 cycles per minute and a 'long tide' potential for the 'fluid within the fluid' of 2.5 cycles per minute, and with the adjacent deeper expression of the Breath of Life about one cycle every 90 seconds. Then the affects of the Field Phenomena (like Earth and Cosmic energy) are "enfolded" in this tuning one cycle every 15 to 20 minutes.

Like the heartbeat, in CranioSacral therapy the **pulse** can be taken at a number of places on the body with a range of harmonics detectable. **The goal of CranioSacral and other manipulative therapies is to facilitate a radiation of this pulse,** which probably relates to Wilhelm Reich's orgone, throughout the rest of the body and its perfect harmonic nesting in the known heart/brain piezoelectrics. Orgone energy is defined as "a complex high frequency/high information density output of **all the cells of the body**". One of its principle bandwidths is in the almost visible

UltraViolet, as evidenced by the **significant UV bursts** accompanying the onset of meiotic and meitotic cellular replicative processes. The cell has accomplished the weaving of the many coarser bandwidths into the refined optical drivers for genetic replication. At such a stage the cell's finest product as information is perceived as orgiastic energy (thus the term orgone).

The Schumann Resonance everywhere present between earth and ionosphere is a **living ringing oscillator** with a harmonic display of significant extremely deep notes spread in a way into a chord of intensities centered and entraining with the brain and body waves. When you observe a graphic representation of the chord of Schumann oscillation within earth's atmosphere it peaks at 7.83, 13.7, 19.6, 25.5, 31.4, 37.3, and 43.2 cycles per second (Hz), with daily variation of about +/- .5 Hz. The manifest vibration of earth at the surface of the lithosphere is 7.5, with between 7.8 and 12 Hz, with an **average value of 10.5 Hz identified as the Alpha rhythm, and 13.7 through 43.2 Hz the Beta brain drivers**. The geometry of the ratio of these frequencies as with any collection of vibrations providing a chord, indicates that **the Schumann rhythm is the natal music of this sphere.** Not only are the major frequencies, spaced at about 5.9 Hz apart, but the frequency divided by its harmonic order gives an average ratio between harmonics of .75.

The brain is a massive source of ELF signals that get transmitted throughout the body through the nervous system, which is sensitive to magnetic fields. Brain waves and natural biorhythms of the body can be entrained by strong external ELF signals, such as the stationary waves of Schumann Resonances. Entrainment, synchronization and amplification promote coherent large-scale activity rather than typical flurries of transient brain waves. Thus, resonant standing waves emerge from the brain, which under the right conditions facilitate internal and external bio-information transfer via ELF electromagnetic waves. These SR waves exhibit non-local character and nearly instant communication capacity. [An example of person-tree communication is given below]

The frequency bands of the brain measured by the EEG (Electroencephalograph) and their wave characteristics are described as follows:

Gamma waves 925-60 Hz) appear to relate to simultaneous processing of information from different brain areas, e.g., involving memory, learning abilities, integrated thoughts or information-rich task processing. Gamma rhythms modulate perception and consciousness, which disappear with anaesthesia. Synchronous activity at about 40 Hz appears involved in binding sensory inputs into the single, unitary objects we perceive.

Beta waves (12-25 Hz) dominate our normal waking state of consciousness when attention is directed towards cognitive tasks and the outside world. Beta is a 'fast' activity, present when we are alert or even anxious, or when engaged in problem solving, judgement, decision making, information processing, mental activity and focus. Nobel Prize winner Sir Francis Crick and other scientists believe the 40 Hz Beta frequency may be key to the act of cognition.

Alpha waves (7-12 Hz) are present during dreaming and light meditation when eyes are closed. As more and more neurons are recruited to this frequency, Alpha waves cycle globally across the whole cortex. This induces deep relaxation, but not quite meditation. In Alpha we begin to access the wealth of creativity that lies just below our conscious awareness. It is the gateway, the entry point that leads into deeper states of consciousness. Alpha waves aid overall mental coordination, calmness, alertness, inner awareness, mind/body integration and learning. Alpha is also the home of the window frequency known as the Schumann Resonance, which propagates with little attenuation around the planet. When we intentionally generate Alpha waves and go into resonance with that Earth frequency, we naturally feel better, refreshed, in tune, in synch. It is, in fact, environmental synchronization.

Theta waves (4-7 Hz) occur most often in sleep but are also dominant in the deepest states of meditation (body asleep/mind awake) and thought (gateway to learning, memory). In Theta, our senses are withdrawn from the external world and focussed on the mindscape-internally originating signals. Theta waves are associated with mystery, an elusive and extraordinary realm we can explore. It is that twilight state which we normally only experience fleetingly as we rise from the depths of Delta upon waking or drifting off to sleep. In Theta we are in a waking dream; vivid imagery flashes before the mind's eye and we are receptive to information beyond our normal conscious awareness. Theta meditation increases creativity, enhances learning, reduces stress and awakens intuition and other extrasensory perception skills.

Delta waves (0-4 Hz) are the slowest but the highest in amplitude. They are generated in deepest meditation and dreamless sleep. Delta waves confer a suspension of external existence and provide the most profound feelings of peace. In addition, **certain frequencies within the Delta range trigger the release of a growth hormone which is beneficial for healing regeneration**. This is why sleep, deep restorative sleep, is so essential to the healing process.

There is a harmonic relationship or resonance between earth and our mind/body. Earth's low-frequency iso-electric field, the magnetic field of earth, and the electromagnetic field which emerges from our body are closely interwoven. Our internal rhythms interact with external rhythms, affecting our balance, REM patterns, health, and mental focus. Schumann Resonance waves probably help regulate our bodies' internal clocks, affecting sleep/dream patterns, arousal patterns, and hormonal secretion (such as *melatonin*). Schumann Resonance fluctuates like brain waves due to geographic location, lightning, solar flares, atmospheric ionization, and daily cycles. The most important daily rhythm is the change in light, called **circadian**, majorly influencing the pineal gland *melatonin* secretion.

The Earth's Geomagnetic field is strongly influenced by the following cycles: the moon's 29.5 day rotation; the earth's own rotation of 365.25 days; sunspot cycles 11 or 22 years; the nutation cycle of 18.6 years; the rotation of the planets of 88 days to 247.7 years; and the galaxy's rotation cycle of 250 million years.

Very important body rhythms, like hormone secretion and dominant nostril exchange, are in the order of 1 to 2 hours. The human EEG is influenced by the sun's electromagnetic oscillation of

10 Hz, while the earth/ionosphere system is resonant at frequencies in the Theta, Alpha, Beta-1 (low or slow) and Beta-2 (high or fast) bands.

NEUROFEEDBACK

The body's bioelectrical domain is geared to thalmocortical generation of rhythmic activity. The degree of this rhythmicity is what is being trained in biofeedback. Rhythmicity manages the entire range of activation and arousal in the bioelectric domain. One role rhythmicity serves may be time-binding, the need to harness the spatially distributed brain electrical activity into that of a single entity. It is believed that the 40 Hz wave serves to connect structures in the cortex, where advanced information processing occurs, and in the thalamus, a lower brain region where complex relay and integrative functions are carried out.

Brainwaves indicate the **arousal dimension**, and arousal mediates a number of conditions as changes in sympathetic and parasympathetic arousal "tune" the nervous system. **Underarousal and suppression of *norepinephrine*** affecting particularly the brain stem leads towards unipolar or reactive depression, attention deficit disorder, chronic pain and insomnia. **Overarousal and overproduction of *norepinephrine*** is linked with anxiety disorders, sleep onset problems, nightmares, hyper-vigil-ance, impulsive behavior, anger/aggression, agitated depression, chronic nerve pain and spasticity. A combination of under-arousal and overarousal causes anxiety and depression as well as ADHD.

Instabilities in certain rhythms can be correlated with tics, obsessive-compulsive disorder, aggressive behavior, rage, bruxism, panic attacks, bipolar disorder, migraines, narcolepsy, epilepsy, sleep apnea, vertigo, tinnitus, norexia-bulemia, suicidal ideation and behavior, PMS, multiple chemical sensitivities, diabetes, hypoglycemia, and explosive behavior.

If people can control their mind patterns in response to generated wave form patterns, they can enter different states of mental being. The mind responds by entraining or attuning to harmonic frequencies in ranges of sound or vibration resonant with its thought patterns. Sound waves are examples of periodicity, of rhythm. Each cycle of a wave is in reality a single pulse of sound. We cannot hear frequencies below our average 8 octave range of 20 Hz to 20,000 Hz, but through the synchronization process of entrainment, where the vibrations of one object will cause the vibrations of another object to oscillate at the same rates, we can perceive them as rhythmic beats.

External rhythms can have a direct effect on the psychology and physiology of the listener. Slower tempos from 40 to 70 beats per minute have been proven to decrease heart and respiratory rate, thereby altering the predominant brainwave patterns. Biofeedback uses binaural beats generated by subtly different frequencies delivered to each ear independently with headphones. When the left channel's pitch is 100 cycles per second and the right channel's pitch is 108 cycles per second, a pulsing *subsonic* 8 Hz tone is heard within the brain itself. These frequencies are generated as both hemispheres of the brain work simultaneously to hear sounds that are **pitch-differed by key mathematical intervals.** The brain waves respond to these oscillating tones by following or entraining to them and both hemispheres begin to work together. Communication between the two sides of the brain is associated with flashes of creativity, insight and wisdom.

Alpha-wave biofeedback is considered a consciousness self-regulation technique, while Alpha-frequency binaural beat stimulation (frequency following response) is a passive management technique where cortical potentials entrain to or resonate at the frequency of the external stimulus. Through the self-regulation of specific cortical rhythms, we begin to control those aspects of consciousness associated with that rhythm. **When the goal is the Alpha brain state, either in meditation or in biofeedback, it means entraining with the primary Schumann Resonance.**

I first encountered the binaural beat with Robert Munroe's 36 binaural guided meditation tapes in the 70s designed to teach out-of-body journeying. His experiences journeying out of his body generated pivotal books, an Institute in VA, and his method of self-induction was so significant that Joseph McMoneagle spent time there in his **remote viewing** training. I never could get Out, but have loaned the Course of tapes to other potential psychonauts.

The ability of the brain to enter and maintain certain frequencies while sleeping may determine the level of health a person experiences. In a large study of individuals suffering the symptoms of Chronic Fatigue (waking up tired, stressed, experiencing symptomatic pain, depression, confused thinking, memory loss, headaches, nervous stomach, or having sleep disorders), patient's measured EEG recordings showed the seven brain wave frequencies to be consistently weaker. These seven frequencies seemed to be guide posts within the subconscious that lead the brain into and out of specific functions necessary for the night's reconstructive process of the body to occur while in the sleep cycle. The weakness or inability to reach and maintain these frequencies related directly to the specific symptom or ailment experienced. Levels of exhaustion from Chronic Fatigue were reduced when individuals were moved to 4 Hz. At 7.5 Hz confused thinking in problem solving was eased. For those whose ailments had manifest into the 4th stage of Chronic Fatigue, where some form of the disease is apparent, a release from negative sensation of their symptoms was experienced when moved to 1.5 Hz.

Increasingly, sophisticated measurement devices expand biofeedback's possibilities. A number of experts are pioneering a new form of EEG training that uses light stimulation to increase the ranges and variability of patient's dominant brain frequencies. The treatment is proving successful with trauma victims whose brains have gotten "stuck" in a pattern of predominantly slow waves associated with underarousal. More and more, biofeedback researchers are discovering that the key is brain flexibility - not a perpetual "Theta state". Biofeedback training seems particularly effective because it gives patients a sense of being in charge, of mastery and self-reliance, over their illness and their health.

Dr Irving Dardik's research on the harmonics of the "waves within waves" of the heart rate variability suggest that the fracticality ratio of .75 is key and clue to virtually all chronic diseases. Marty Wuttke found that in thousands of clinically documented case he was able to facilitate sustained elimination of addiction (also ADD) by steering the EEG brainwave series of wavelengths into a geometry of embedding or recursion, creating a sustainable contiguous EEG harmonic series. When EEG harmonics enter or are balanced into a broad spectrum of perfectly nested PHI ratio series, addiction goes away because the cellular thrust for ECK or charge in stasis (ecstasy) becomes self-generating and requires no substance abuse. After feedback, the excess of the high frequency EEG has smoothed out to a more even and contiguous harmonic series, completing a situation where a charge cascade between harmonics becomes sustainable.

Once ECK in stasis is achieved, Dan Winter says, "it is not interrupted by harmonics which don't fit the series embedding. Complete the fractal and you have sustainable charge and ability to effectively electrically embed environment. Essentially, the charge envelope of nesting perfected in the wave-length of brainwaves creates apparently a container for sustaining charge-waves non-destructively. Thus, when the EEG harmonics enter into a perfectly nested series, at that point addiction goes away because ECK or Charge in Stasis (Ecstacy) becomes self-generating and requires no substance abuse. The principle is that again the geometry of perfect embedding or recursion is the key to self-awareness."

Along with the brain's complex EEG wave patterns, this model connects the spectrum of heart harmonics (EKG) with perceived emotional states and **extends the influence of intentional internal vibration out into the apparent universe.** The Schumann resonance of the planet is thus often called our collective heartbeat. The musical octaves expressed in its peak frequencies have an average ratio between harmonics of .75. **An excellent expression of the Schumann resonance as a living ringing oscillator is shown in these spectrum analyses of a tree** (below), charted from the output of a biological capacitive probe designed by Prof Phil Callahan with charge amplifier and compared after interaction with intense human emotion, found on Dan Winter's very extensive site on this subject at www.soulinvitation.com.

As picked up by sensors on an oak tree embedded in the Schumann resonance, there is first shown an average 'being there' ratio between harmonics of .685. Peaks on the below graphed wavelengths are around those of earth energy, with scattered wavelengths between and a strong very low activity Theta/Delta/ zero wave (arrow), followed by fairly strong Alpha and 4 declining intensities of Beta (clearer in upper part of the analysis.

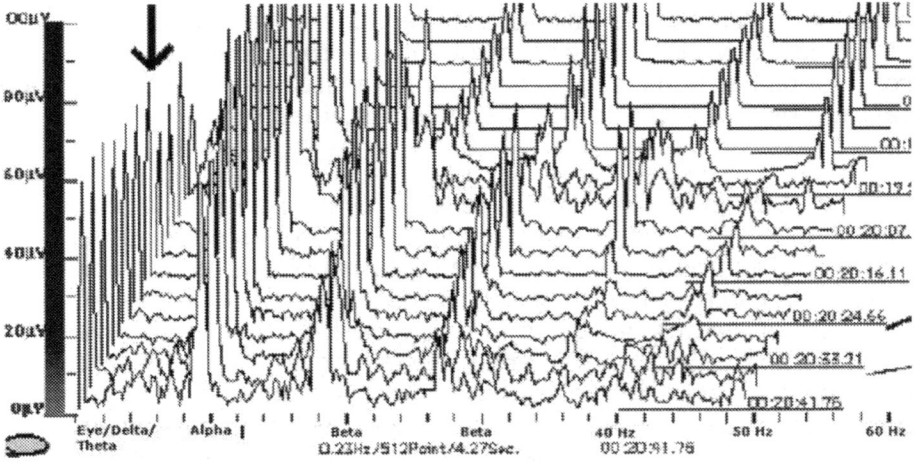

The ratio of .685 between beats may be approaching .618, which is PHI or the Golden Mean (literally the feeling of LOVE) and is the mathematical perfection that allows systems to be harmonically embedded within systems – the only 'angle' at which a wave can re-enter itself without destroying itself.

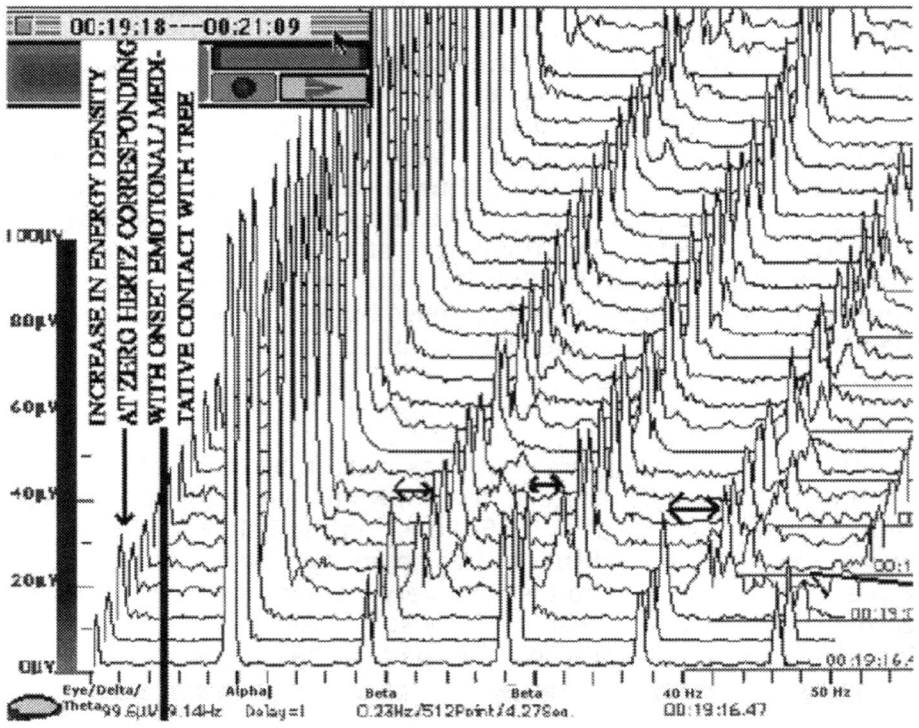

INCREASE IN ENERGY DENSITY AT ZERO HERTZ CORRESPONDING WITH ONSET EMOTIONAL/ MEDITATIVE CONTACT WITH TREE

After human meditative contact with the tree, the EEG impression on the tree is clear, as zero/low decreases, Alpha soars, and three peaks of Beta get more clearly organized, with more distinct gaps between them.

The brain as an oscillator that creates self-awareness by recursion in its own resonance can now learn for earth. In this fashion, our collective emotional magnetism can add to the recursive nesting glue which holds the **tectonic song lines** together. Dan Winter says that "this skill to choose how to radiate magnetics by emoting coherently (like a laser) is the most powerful tool we have to save our genepool." We have a "maximum need to create global coherent emotion; **the Schumann resonance of the planet is often called our collective heartbeat for a reason**".

The average male voice **resonates at B flat 120 Hz, 2 octaves below C and 2 octaves above Beta brain activity. The average** female speaking voice **of 250 Hz is about an octave higher. The** voice range **is about three octaves, from 85 Hz to 1100 Hz.**

Humans hear **wavelengths as low as the vibrations of their brains and bodies (20 Hz) for a span of 8 octaves to 20,000 Hz.**

Cats' hearing **starts at 60 Hz (the 'sound' of Alternating Current at 60 cycles a second) and spans 10 octaves to an octave and a half above humans at 65,000 Hz. They make sounds only in the two octaves above G above C.**

Bats' voice **starts in our highest octave 10,000 Hz and monitors about two and a half octaves beyond, to 120,000 Hz. They can hear in the same range, as well as three octaves below their vocal range -- down into the human vocal range at 1000 Hz.**

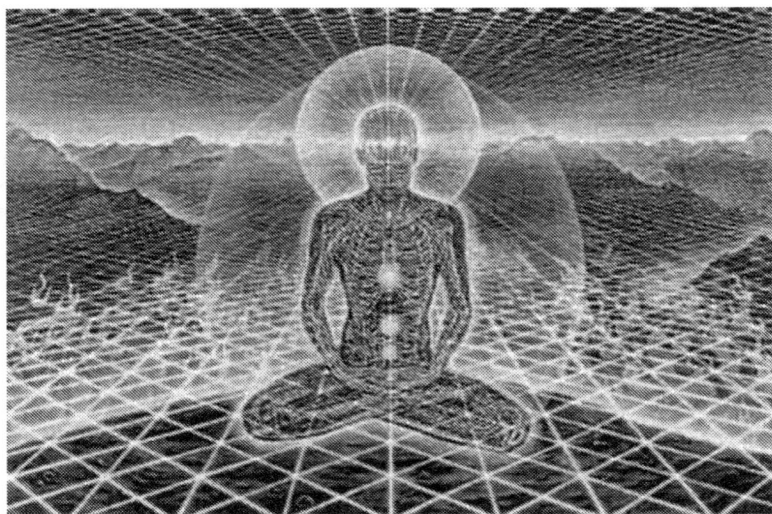

Natural Pranic Health

There are three principle sources of prana: air prana through the act of respiration, solar prana through exposure to sunlight, and ground prana through our feet as we walk around and from the food we eat, an indirect way of obtaining prana that ultimately comes from air, earth, and sun. Prana is another name for energy. Prana is remarkably powerful and resilient, yet it is also delicate. Prana can be used to relieve serious health problems - even projected over great distances without losing its strength or effectiveness - but your prana can also be diminished or weakened by many factors, including your beliefs, emotions, attitudes, inhibitions, and traumatic memories, the food you eat, the people you associate with, where you work and live, how you work and live, what you say, what you think, and how you react to the general level of stress in your life. It is also affected by the radiations and toxins in your environment.

Our environment is literally out of tune with Nature itself. There is an urgent need for us to understand how everything alive responds to the most subtle changes in magnetic and electro-magnetic fields surrounding and interpenetrating us. Serious at-tention must now be paid to the possible biological role of standing waves in the atmosphere so that we do not overlook the import-ance of oscillations in Nature that may be central to consciousness and life itself. The living of life depends upon the balance of two environmental signals described in ancient Chinese teachings as the **YIN** (feminine) weaker geomantic waves coming from below - from within the planet - and the **YANG** (masculine) relatively stronger 3 Hz to 300 Hz Schumann wave surrounding our planet.

IMMUNITY BOOSTING

The body's own immune system if sufficiently strengthened and boosted by natural means, can resist or weather an attack by any biological organism. To learn, is how to treat and resist disease conditions naturally, without the need for drugs or so-called 'vaccines'.

The body's health is directly related to what you ingest. With modern supermarket food **devitalized by contaminants and by its processing by food manufacturing and food delivery,** the value of researching and taking action to enable one's proper nutrition cannot be emphasized enough. Organic fresh raw foods possess forms of energy and vibrations not currently understood by orthodox science. If you open your intention to psi energy, you can dowse for the 'vital force' of food. Raw foods also contain digestive enzymes that cooked and processed foods lack. The **digestive enzymes that Nature provides accompanying raw fruit, vegetable, or meat is the perfect match for that particular food.** If those enzymes aren't in the food that you eat, your body has to make them, requiring energy and additional nutrients that deplete your energy resources. Many researchers who study those elements that contribute to longevity feel that **the human body has a limited capacity and store of enzyme production over a life time. When your enzyme producing capacity expires, you expire!**

Vitamins and minerals are most bio-available in Nature's form. Adding de-Natured vitamins back into vitamin deficient food through fortification will not give you the equivalent quality of bio-activity of vitamins and their inter-relatedness as originally provided by nature. That nutritional deficiency is quite common in the US, despite the abundance of ready and waiting food, indicates that fortified foods cannot provide the equivalent nutrition and bio-activity as provided by Nature in its original raw food state.

We are all exposed to anti-nutrients through food and water that antagonize the body's intake and its generation of health. Some anti-nutrients bind to make necessary nutrients useless, others tie-up the enzymes needed for digestion and other body functions, some cause nutrients including those the body makes to be excreted more rapidly or create a greater need for certain nutrients. Many anti-nutrients have either a direct or indirect affect on immune function. Whatever you can do to reduce your exposure to anti-nutrients will be helpful in preventing recurrent illness. Sugar, food coloring, processed fats, additives like BHT, and most of the 3,000 or so allowed additives to food beyond nature's wisdom often act as anti-nutrients. **American agriculture uses 4.5 pounds of pesticides for every man woman and child in the country each year!** (you know the size of a 5 pound bag of sugar) The adverse effects of these chemicals are more of a problem than most would imagine.

See pages 133 to 137 on Supplementation of Nutrients.

SUGAR lowers immunity, decreasing the ability of white blood cells to engulf and destroy ever present bacteria. Sugar is added to almost every packaged food such that **the average adult consumes more than 150 pounds of sugar each year** - 14 times more than 100 years ago and far too much for our bodies to handle. Refined **disaccharide sucrose sugar is not what you want**. Fresh fruit is the best sweet source **for fructose, the natural monosaccharide, handled differently by the body**. Otherwise, you just have to know the dimensions of your sugar addiction and do what you are willing in order to support your immune system - the key to your health. **The no calorie sweetener SPLENDA, of dextrose, maltodextrin, and sucralose sugars seems the best choice for sweetening.**

ZINK LEVELS are depleted by sugar, and with their **decline the sense of taste declines as well, creating the need for more flavor - or added sugar.** Developing addiction to taste perception drives the manufacturing market. They know what they are doing and why. I take 50 mg daily, not more than 100 mg.

Excessive consumption of **COW'S MILK** is often one of the major factors contributing to susceptibility to common infections. There's plenty of proof of this. An 86 year old German study of 49,362 children born in 1890 concluded, "Further statistics show of those fed on mother's milk one in thirteen died, while of those brought up by hand (bottle-fed), one out of every two died." This was well before pharmacy and pesticides. In "MILK IS GOOD FOR _____" by MD Robert M Kradjian: "Among children the problems were allergy, ear and tonsils infections, bedwetting, asthma, intestinal bleeding, nephritis, colic, childhood diabetes." "In adults the problems seemed centered more around heart disease, arthritis, allergy, sinusitis, and the more serious questions of leukemia, lymphoma, cancer (colon, lung, prostate, breast, ovarian, rectal)." "Even multiple sclerosis. Osteoporosis, and cataracts have been associated with cow's milk consumption."

I haven't drunk milk for decades. Giving up dairy **BUTTER**, though, was a problem solved some time ago by delicious 100% vegan **SOY BUTTER** that is a perfect substitute.

THE FLEXIBLE VEGETARIAN DIET

Albert Einstein said, "Nothing will benefit human health and increase the chances for survival of life on earth as much as the evolution to a vegetarian diet." The vegetarian menu is a powerful and pleasant way to achieve good health. The vegetarian eating pattern is based on a wide variety of foods that are satisfying, delicious, and healthful. Avoiding meat and poultry, some 'vegetarians' may eat fish for protein. Some include dairy products and eggs (lacto-ovo vegetarians) The vegan diet eschews all meats, eggs, and dairy and is the healthiest diet to reduce risk of a broad range of health concerns.

Vegetarian meals are typically low in saturated fats and usually contain little or no cholesterol - found in animal products. Many studies show that replacing animal protein with plant protein lowers blood cholesterol levels even if fat in the diet stays the same. Heart disease is uncommon in vegetarians. When patients with high blood pressure begin a vegetarian diet many are able to eliminate their need for medication.

This is just a small excerpt you might like to know from the "Vegetarian Starter Kit":

1. Percentage of pesticide residues in the US diet supplied by grains: 1%

2. Percentage of pesticide residues in the US diet supplied by Fruits: 4%

3. Percentage of pesticide residues in the US diet supplied by dairy products: 23%

4. Percentage of pesticide residues in the US diet supplied by meat: 55%

5. Pesticide contamination of breast milk from meat eating mothers vs. non-meat eating: 35 times higher

6. What the USDA tells us: meat is inspected.

7. Percentage of slaughtered animals inspected for residues of toxic chemicals including dioxin and DDT: less than 0.00004% (That's four hundred thousandth)

FIBER

Fiber is essential in the diet to keep things moving, and because foods like **fruit, vegetables, legumes and grains (oats, wheat, rice, barley, etc.) are high in vitamins, trace minerals, and essential fatty acids**. If intestinal contents move too slowly, toxic by-products of digestion and bacterial fermentation remain in the bowel too long and are reabsorbed back into the body. Over time this can contribute to illness. With a low fiber diet, parasites such as *giardia* attack more readily, contributing to immune suppression, poor digestion, food allergies, and numerous other problems. The high intake of dietary fiber is associated with a significantly reduced risk of weight problems, abdominal obesity, hyper-tension, and high cholesterol and triglycerides.

Processed food usually removes what you are eating it for. Take WHEAT, for example: Almost all essential nutrients are bound in the germ portion of the grain. During milling, the germ is separated from the endosperm. The germ is sold separately as wheat germ (long known as a high nutrient food), while the endosperm is further milled to make flour. Milling of whole grain to make refined flour results in loss of 85% of the *magnesium,* 86% of the *manganese,* 40% of the *chromium*, 78% of the *zink*, 86% of the *cobalt*, 48% of the *molybdenum,* and 68% of the *copper*, in addition to comparable losses of *selenium*, vitamin E and essential fatty acids. Morover, heavy metals such as c*admium* (which are concentrated in the endosperm) remain in the flour - unfortunately, the body's antagonist to *cadmium, zink*, has been removed. Since nutrients are required to properly utilize all categories we consume, **the intake of refined food leads to a gradual deficiency of nutrients**. A strong argument for the use of whole-grain products.

JUICING

Juicing adds to the benefits if vegetables and fruit, allowing the important nutrients and phytochemicals found in plants to be absorbed more easily and in greater quantity. When foods are cooked, enzymes essential for digestion and absorption of food, for conversion of food into body tissue, and for the production of energy at the cellular level can be destroyed. That is why raw foods and juices are so important. Buying commercial juice you must avoid sweetness and additives and anything heat-treated to extend shelf life which can destroy nutrients.

RECOMMENDED DIET

For those of you looking for a suggested diet, the vegetarian logic suggests the following:

*   Consume a diet that focuses on whole, unprocessed foods (whole grains, legumes, vegetables, fruits, seeds, etc.)
*   Reduce (or eliminate, if possible) your intake of refined sugar.
*   Drink at least 8 to 10 glasses of water daily.
*   Avoid animal products, with the possible exception of cold water fish (salmon, mackerel, herring, halibut, etc.).
*   Eliminate dairy products, excessive caffeine, and alcohol.
*   Avoid soft drinks completely.
*   Avoid white bread and refined flour products. They are devoid of essential nutrients, including omega-3 essential fatty acids and others.
*   Avoid margarine and all commercial cooking oils. Use Butter and Organic cold pressed Olive oil instead, or the new soy butters that taste even better than butter
*   Consume organic Flax Seed Oil and cold fish oil (MAX EPA) daily. Hemp oil is even better balanced .
*   Consume Miso soup, kelp, and shitake mushrooms regularly.
*   Brown Rice is better than white rice.
*   Buy organic foods (especially produce) whenever possible.
*   Get regular exercise.
*   Perform a relaxation exercise (deep/focused breathing, meditation, tai chi, visualization, prayer, etc.) 10 to 15 minutes each day.

WATER

Water is an essential part of a healthy diet. **Dehydration is an extraordinarily common cause of an astounding number of diseases.** Tea, coffee, alcohol, and manufactured beverages contain de-hydration agents that get rid of the water they are dissolved in plus some water from the reserves of the body. The body must receive its daily need of water. **If you listen to and don't suppress its cries for water** - indicators of regional thirst and drought in the body - you can respond to your own needs appropriately, perhaps with 8-10 glasses of water daily, and more if you are suffering from an illness. Structured water makes an additional big difference to the veritable DNA of every cell in your body. See The Geometry of Water in All-That-Is Waving.

FLUORIDE absolutely must be avoided. Avoid ingesting fluoride. Among other places, fluoride is found in commercial soft drinks, bottled or canned ice tea, and tap water. Fluoride impairs will power and clarity of thought, which makes one more susceptible to microwave mind programming signals. It is part of the mind control program, converting us into obedient receivers of controlling microwave wavelengths that permeate every nook and cranny of the country.

COFFEE FOR SHORT TERM MEMORY

MRI studies after consumption of 100 mg of caffeine (2 small cups) revealed heightened memory, attention, and reaction time. Coffee turns out to be America's most abundant source of protect-ive anti-oxidants, with Green Tea (3 cups) and black tea (2 1/2 cups) next. Two cups a day is good memory protection. Not late in the day and with extra water to balance its dehydration affect.

AVOID SPRING MATTRESSES. Springs are like antennas and focus electromagnetic and ELF energy into your body while you sleep. Since 1960 they have been included in (MKDELTA) CIA "programming behavior and attitudes in the general public" The best purchase I have made for my spinal health has been an expensive memory-foam 8" mattress, developed for the space program, which supports the body evenly related to its weight pressure and keeps the spine aligned in any position.

SALT

The colloidal special metals from organic sea water have properties of both physical metals and spiritual etheric metals. These colloidal metals are of such small size in Newtonian and Einsteinian physics that they are able to retain a phase-shifting capability between Planckian quantum spiritual physics within their electron structure. By using pure dried sea salt as Europe still does, one is able to acquire a minimal amount of these naturally dried **Orbitally Rearranged Molecular Elements** (ORMEs) with both physical and spiritual properties. America has gone to white man's industrial by-product salt and this could be the entire reason for the massive increase in cancer within the American population.

Meanwhile the German alchemists of the Black Government have magnetized ORMEs to provide vehicle structure, levitation, warp speed pressure movement, and invisibility [see <u>Salt of the Earth, Sea, and Sky</u> in <u>All-That-Is Waving</u>].

One can drink these sea salts back in saline concentration straight or within vegetable (V8) drinks. The rate of assimilation of these special valency metals is lower, but the entire periodic range of ORME metals is gained across the board for absolute assimilation. I have been assuming adequate trace metal intake since the alternative community switched to sea salt in the 60s, but of course that is not what you get in any processed food. Because salts work together, **your diet should include five times as much *potassium* as *sodium*. *Potassium* supplements should balance out your *sodium* habit.** The unknowing American diet/taste usually contains five times as much *sodium* as *potassium,* so the *potassium* ratio must be adjusted. *Potassium* and *sodium* also have relation to *calcium*'s 2:1 relationship with *magnesium* (math that needs factoring!). Current guidelines call for 4,700 mg/day. A proper diet could include 8,000 mg of Potassium/day - the level we evolved to eat. Potassium is remarkably effective at lowering blood pressure, preventing kidney stones and heart arrhythmias and, unless you have kidney disease, one of those things you just can't get enough of.

FATTY ACIDS

The fatty acids in fish may help ward off depression. benefiting not just the heart but also a range of psychiatric problems from bipolar disorder and schizophrenia to depression, ADHD, Alzheimers and borderline personality disorder. It is like neuronal fertilizer to help build cell membranes, boost levels of serotonin and increase the number of connections between neurons. It stimulates bone metabolism, laying down the matrix upon which calcium and other minerals are deposited.

VITAMIN D AND THE SUN'S WAVELENGTHS

It is almost impossible to get enough Vitamin D from diet.

Until the mid 1990's it was believed that the kidneys make the body's entire supply of activated Vitamin D from the 25-Vitamin D created by the liver out of the Vitamin D made in the skin after sun exposure and, to a lesser extent, from foods that supply Vitamin D. The supply from the kidneys that was thought to contribute to bone health is actually small and doesn't change however much 25-Vitamin D there is in the bloodstream. It is now understood that a variety of cells have this ability to activate Vitamin D, including the breast, prostate, colon, brain, skin and probably most other tissues and cells, where it is converted and used on the spot without increasing the activated Vitamin D in the blood stream, making difficulties for scientists to detect the connections between sun exposure and Vitamin D.

We now know that sun exposure has a role in preventing auto-immune diseases such as multiple sclerosis, rheumatoid arthritis and type 1 diabetes, osteoporosis and that it promotes bone health. Vitamin D is best known for its effects on the bones. Discovering that cells throughout the body can activate Vitamin D **is a major breakthrough in Vitamin D research. Also discovered is that not only the**

brain makes 'feel good' endorphins, when exposed to ultraviolet radiation, the skin also makes beta endorphins.

All of us over age one need to get at least 1000 IU of Vitamin D every day. Most of us need only a few minutes a day sun exposure during the summer months to maintain healthy Vitamin D levels throughout the year! About half of the amount of UVB exposure it would take to begin to turn your particular skin pink equals approximately 1000 IU of Vitamin D. Vitamin D is stored in your body fat and released in winter when you need it. Excess fat stores make Vitamin D less bioavailable. 1000 IU or 25,000 nanograms can also be found in a pound of cooked eel or 40 eggs, 10 cups of fortified milk (with the danger of too much calcium), 10 oz salmon or mackerel, 7 1/2 lbs of fortified dried cereal. How about anchovies? Aside from fish, dietary sources of Vitamin D are few and far between.

There is no clear-cut research linking Vitamin D deficiency with flu prevention - since research dollars go towards studying new profitable drugs, but you have a lot to gain and nothing to lose by taking a little extra Vitamin D in the winter, especially in the North. Seasons, geography, and skin tone as well as hospitalization (up to 80% of nursing home patients are deficient) contribute to Vitamin D deficiencies. Dr Whitaker recommends a concerted effort to get about 15 minutes of unprotected (no sun screen) sun exposure several times a week. If you are dark-skinned or live at a higher altitude, you'll require more time in the sun for optimal Vitamin D-25 production.

Neither Vitamin D rich foods nor supplements will cause your body to produce the feel-good substances such as beta-endorphins and *serotonin*, which create the feeling of well being you feel after being in the sun (or using a proper UVB tanning facility). Unlike Vitamin D supplements, which can cause toxicity especially if overdone with children, sun exposure cannot cause toxicity.

We have been *indoctrinated* with an entire bogus construct concerning sunlight. Dr William Campbell Douglas says "Let's put it right up front so there's no confusion:

1)   The sun does not cause melanoma or any other form of fatal cancer. Dermatologists warn that it does, but they have no scientific basis for the assertion. The real fact is, it is more likely that a lack of adequate sunlight is a strong factor to the development of melanoma. The sun is your friend, but like any good thing, using a little self-control makes it even better.

2)   Sunscreen is detrimental to good health and should be avoided. There has been a dramatic rise in melanoma coupled with the use of sun blocking oils.

3)   Sunglasses are also bad for your health unless you wear the full spectrum variety. The sun does not cause cataracts or other visual problems. The infra-red rays from incandescent light bulbs are probably the main cause of cataracts. Use full spectrum fluorescent lights in your home or office."

For a wavelength to 'burn' it means over-exposure to the tolerances of the body for that specific wave-length. Our body can stand great quantities of and variability of exposure to radiation in the ranges of the visible spectrum. At both edges of this visible wavelength band is where intolerances, particularly in the epidermal layer, reveal themselves. Wavelengths of ultraviolet not normally visible 'burn' the skin when it's too much, at the same time the invisible wavelengths of ultra-violet are an essential nutrient in the body's production of Vitamin D.

Melanomas tend to appear on parts of the body not especially exposed to sunlight. They tend to be thicker and more advanced when found on hidden areas of the body. They can be obscured by hair and by a lack of pigmentation. My mother's upper-thigh melanoma in her 70's she said was as large as half a grapefruit.

Almost all the contributory damage to the skin that might induce non-melanoma skin cancer from the sun occurs in childhood and early adulthood – my doctor said the many

basal cell carcinoma skin cancers I burned off from the second epidermal layer of my face with something called *Efudex* after he had frozen off several over years take 26 years to develop. Thus, people over 70 do not need to have concern for anything other than getting enough UVB sun to achieve and maintain healthy Vitamin D levels, which is harder to do the older you get, and are much more likely to die from Vitamin D deficiency-related hip fracture due to osteoporosis than from skin cancer.

Again, it is almost impossible to get enough Vitamin D from diet. **Dr Whitaker says that every physician should recommend Vitamin D supplements. For healthy people with adequate sun exposure, 800 to 1,000 IU of vitamin D3 (*cholecalciferol*) per day should suffice. North of the 40th parallel, 2,000 IU/day from late Fall to early Spring, assuming summer exposure dropping back to 800 to 1,000 IU/day. Individuals with dark skin are at risk with lower levels of Vitamin D because they may require up to ten times more sun exposure to produce the same amount of Vitamin D-25 as those with fairer complexions.**

THE NUTRITIVE ULTRA-VIOLET WAVELENGTH BAND

When I suddenly became six feet tall in the sixth grade, and because my last name begins with 'S' which always had located me in the back of the classroom, I started a slumping down which is still apparent in my stance in order to not stand out, and had to get glasses because **I didn't want to see** my slowly-oncoming adolescence. In my 50's I was able to discard those glasses by letting full-spectrum wavelengths of light bathe my eyes.

Seven out of ten persons wear glass on their faces, all of us ride in conveyances sheathed in glass, and our houses boast lots of it, as all of these glass shields cut us off from our only access to the rays of natural sunlight. A century or so ago, none of this was true. Nor did people slather themselves with protective ointments, don sunglasses and hope to slowly develop a tan for cosmetic purposes, rather than enjoying modest sun to accomplish some of those same aims and, as well, **soaking up the full and necessary spectrum of natural light while shaded by hats, trees and structures. What all of society has lost, to the detriment of its collective immune system, is one of the most important components in human body mainten-ance, access to the necessary ultra-violet wavelengths.**

Consider what science actually reports about light as well as oxygen. Though the news is frequently concerned about the ozone layer, the actual fact is that there is now 15-19% *less* oxygen available in the air we breathe than there was just 50-100 years ago, with 10 percent of that loss occurring in the last 30 years. As well, we receive 15% less light, including the important ultra-violet light component, now striking the earth and contained in the ambient light around us. This information is found in Smithsonian (Kitt's Peak) US reported data, also from analysis of Antarctic boring, and even in the air trapped in builder's spirit levels of past periods and similar trapped-air sources. There is a relationship we mammals have to oxygen that relates directly to our health and, especially, to our immune systems. Significantly less oxygen is available to us now than was to our grandparents. I am leaving aside the implications of the probably increased presence of carbon dioxide, levels of which also help regulate body exchange and circadian functioning (and promote plants) and the surely increased 78% nitrogen (which plants also like), and the known and unknown pollutants. All of which makes it a real fact that it is a lot darker out there than it used to be, we have to work harder for our oxygen, and these significant changes have had wide-reaching biological affects, particularly on our immune systems.

The wavelengths of **the Ultraviolet spectrum nutrient**, which have been cut off from the body as we have gone to living behind glass, are a complex subject of examination. This is because **our body, in fact, expects to receive the full spectrum of the sun's gift to this planet and languishes in various ways when it is separated from it**. We all know about the relationship between UV, the production of Vitamin D, and the absorption of calcium. (What we don't know is that, even with sticking the Vitamin D into the calcium milk, those elderly, living separated off from most of us, still mostly don't absorb that calcium without receiving *some* of the necessary UV wavelengths from ambient sunlight.) When we connect up some of the things we know about wavelengths, parents all know about the irradiation of newborns with blue-light wavelength to prevent bilirubin jaundice. They've learned about SAD (Seasonal Adjustment Syndrome) and the necessity for brightness of light to trigger, via the pineal gland, the necessary body-rhythm adjustments to the seasons. Less well known is that human cholesterol levels also drop under the influence of sunlight.

Our trying to understand SAD provides instruction about the interface between the eyes, as receptors of nutrients that come in the form of wavelengths, and with pineal functions which control *serotonin*, the brain's "feel good" transmitter. **Serotonin production is directly related to the duration of exposure to sunlight** (Lancet 2002). There are great differences in different entities' relationships to the light deprivation that accompanies winter. Some people are particularly hard hit by light deprivation and may be clinically described as "depressed", as one in five is statistically described. They manifest longer sleeping periods, increased appetites and cravings for carbohydrates, and often weight gain. This malady is seasonal in its manifestation, more common in northern latitudes, affecting five percent of the population and twice as many women as men. In these cases, Dr Julian Whitaker says, "light therapy is so helpful that I would recommend that anyone suffering with depression, even if it is not seasonal, try it. It is a much safer and natural way of raising mood-enhancing *serotonin* levels than Prozac and other drugs." Next best, he recommends that "**full spectrum home and workplace lighting relieves eyestrain, brightens mood and improves other aspects of health.**"

Until recently, the use of light as a nutrient in photobiological medicine and phototherapy has been largely suppressed by the "Four Horsemen of the Apothecary": (1) the drug companies, (2) The FDA,

(3) the researchers who work for the drug companies, and (4) the medical journal industry that works in collusion with the drug companies to brainwash us all. With the advent of the new age of pestilence, with new disease syndromes such as AIDS, CFS, Herpes, Palestine Syndrome, chlamidia, plus the counterattack of microbes we thought we had conquered, light therapy to enhance the immune system should become the treatment of choice for infectious diseases.

Wavelength aspects of cytoluminescent therapy work as follows: bacterial and viral cells contain at least 5 times as much of two photosensitive amino acids as do healthy red and white blood cells and thus have proportionately greater photoactive sensitivity. Diseased cells are characteristically smaller in size than healthy cells, with thinner shells, and absorb 5 times as much introduced photonic light energy as do their healthy counterparts.The killed and marked cells are eliminated, as is routine, by normal body-blood editing functions. Different wavelengths have different affects. The section on Body Energies covers light communicating within the body and more about the effect of different colors of light.

In one form or another, ultraviolet irradiation of the blood has been in continuous use by physicians for over 50 years. It has been approved by the FDA for the treatment of cutaneous T-cell lymphoma. It is safe, effective in a broad range of diseases, without side effects, and relatively inexpensive. One method is to withdraw only 10cc's of whole blood with a quartz syringe (at 5 million per cubic millimeter, that's about 50 billion red blood corpuscles), exposing it for 3 minutes to ultraviolet light and other wavelengths of the electromagnetic spectrum 100 times the energy of ambient sunlight, while simultaneously increasing the oxygen level in the body with a slow hydrogen peroxide (.015% solution) therapy-enhancing drip. Light activating psoralin (8 MOP) or certain photosensitive amino acids, herbs, dyes, or porphyrin derivatives in the blood can also increase the photodynamic effect. An average increased blood oxygen absorption of 50% can be expected thirty days after such irradiation. Another method of treatment since the 1940s is a continuous flow IV system irradiating the blood as it is pumped behind a pure quartz glass window (remember, regular glass, as on our faces, doesn't let the ultraviolet wavelengths through).

While we suspect that the eyes take in most of our sensory information and are a gateway to the mind; we need also to know that eyes are an important *gateway to the body*. The nervous system and the endocrine system are *directly* stimulated and regulated by ultraviolet light wavelengths which are received by specific photoreceptors in the eye which have direct connection to the <u>hypothalamus gland</u> of the brain (nervous system, hormonal balance, energy balance, sleep, growth, reproduction, emotional balance), the <u>pituitary gland</u> (metabolism, hormones) and to the <u>pineal gland</u> (circadian rhythms, aging, melatonin, the "third eye"). **Metabolism and glandular activities are, thus, directly regulated by receiving the lower end of the visual spectral environme**nt. (Not to mention microwave wavelengths near and far <u>outside </u>of the visual spectrum, which we are beginning to realize may affect us considerably also.) All of this explains why my guru in the UV matter, Dr. John Nash Ott, predicted in his books of the 60's and 70's that this was a society that would be visited by **ever-increasing diseases of the immune system**. He knew that we had cut ourselves off from the UV nutrient by glass, fear, and fashion, but I don't think he also knew that *less and less of it was ambiently available*. (To worry, as they do, about *increasing* ultraviolet and the ozone layer, indeed!) In Ott's 60's no one then yet knew much even about hepatitis and, at that time, much less about the over-all malevolently created disease of the immune system (AIDS) now manifesting in countless garbs. While I believe the reception of UV wavelengths through the eyes is intimately associated with the immune system, the circadian biological clock, aging, sleep and dreaming, etc., as above, it is the affect upon the muscles of the eye and one's seeing of the world and how I applied this information with John Ott's support and encouragement upon which I wish also to focus (sic).

I used this UV healing information to deal with my major manifestation of up-tight maturation which medicine labels "diseased" vision. I "nearsighted" for almost 40 years. A most significant activity of the UV spectrum range as a nutrient is its part as major stimulus to the ciliary muscle which, basically, controls your vision. Wavelengths, of course, are intrinsic to everything! The ciliary muscle is a donut of eye muscle from the center of which the lens and the iris are suspended. As one steps out of the cave into brighter light, UV wavelengths are expected to trigger that ciliary muscle into closing down the iris (instead of blocking sunglasses). A healthy muscle which has not atrophied into a set position from living behind glass and sunglasses has a full range of possible settings from contracted small to totally-relaxed and fully extended. In order to expand (get bigger), a lens-holding complete donut circle of ciliary muscle has **relaxation** as its only choice. Being "up tight" or squinting **will not** relax (expand) it and, indeed, works against it. If the ciliary muscle complex in maturation is held to rigid dimensions through disuse and atrophy induced by prosthetic manipulation, it cannot relax. One simply cannot see at a distance, then, for it is the extension of the edge lens diameter and the flattening of the aqueous lens that accommodates the focusing at a distance. You can test this UV contraction-trigger yourself by exiting a house into brighter outside light and mirror-viewing both of your eyes with one situated behind plain glass and the other "exposed". The iris of the exposed eye that receives the ambient UV trigger will close slightly more than the one located behind glass, however conditioned that iris has become to it's prosthesis in the form of glasses, sunglasses, or simply from living always behind glass.

Visual acuity (the ability to see detail) and depth-of-field (the ability to see clearly and simultaneously things at different distances) are influenced by pupil diameter. The smaller the pupil diameter the better visual acuity and depth-of-field. Many of the eye's responses to light are determined by the rods that can even (after 1/2 hour dark adjustment) perceive movement in the dark. The rods have their peak response at blue-green 509 nanometers, optimized in full-spectrum lighting and when stepping out of the cave. The eye's responses to light are determined by the rods (scotopic night vision) not the cones (photopic - day vision). Lamps with color temperatures of illumination of 5000 K and higher can improve pupil size and achieve the same lighting task performance to replace incandescent lamps of lower UV and color temperature.

In my 50's, over 20 years ago, on my way to three weeks of winter camping in the sun-drenched Virgin Islands, I realized that precise vision was not necessary in paradise. I could discard my glasses and be an Ott disciple in the natural living style the 70's were promoting. My glasses of almost 40 years were prosthesis for astigmatic Left 20/260 Right 20/200 with closest (reading) focus possible then in my 'middle age' only beyond about 2 feet away. Almost everyone's eye strengths are imbalanced and each eye takes on different functions in their over-all tandem sterioptical relationship to depth perception and focus. I was 50 years old making that decision on that 14-passenger plane out of old San Juan airport, and having trouble trying to thread a needle. "Everybody gets farsighted with age", medicine says, *reporting what it observes as though it were causative.* Prescription sunglasses were in vogue then and I had indeed bought some, and loved them (I liked the brown world better than the blue). Expensive chameleon glass lenses were just arriving then also. **I didn't *have* to see, when I discarded my prostheses, but I intended to**! The only Affirmation (another 70's thing) I used **was to consistently tell myself "I relax into seeing**". Any straining to see, like squinting, tenses the very muscles which must relax in order to focus. In six months, I passed the eye test and got the restriction taken off of my MA driver's license, and in 2 years the haloes around lights I had seen for years without glasses at night had stopped (I'm now hearing about these haloes reported by people who have had laser surgery). My 77-year old right eye focuses well at an optimal 29" up to about 9" away -- so much for the aging myth about far-sighting (reading problems) being inevitable. Five years before, a bungee cord escaping from my construction roof rack scratched my left eye and had me back at the UMass Kaiserated eye guy's place for examination. He knew my left eye's 20/260 history as he tested the recently attacked left eye at 20/15 on three visits without comment. You can imagine that I commented. Subsequently, he still wrote a longish admonition in the Kaiser newsletter about the dangers of UV and the need to always have proper protective sunglasses (which they furnish, in vogue).

Which brings me to the core of this number and the reason for this "personal testimony". What I'm talking about here is actually an exercise plan, something that's quite popular these days. I've done workshops and lots of proselytizing for natural eye health but have had only a handful of disciples. Teaching a workshop at GAYLA twice got one man to try it and my Tibetan-meditation friend Thom did it for a year with only medium results. Yet I know it works because it worked for me and *it makes complete bodysense*. Work out a nutritional and radical wavelength exercise plan for your own eyes and discard the prosthesis! A few week's living outside in paradise, when you don't need to see precisely, helps a great deal. This can accomplish deep levels of change rather than graduating you to a stronger pair of visual crutches. Otherwise, 20 mid-day minutes a day in the ambient should feed you.

Two other comments about this exercise program: **"Ambient light" means that light which surrounds you and does not necessitate ever being in direct sun**. Sunglasses are the worst possible prosthesis to put on your body – a healthy iris will close down adequately to serve aborigine and urban dweller equally well, with the only need for protection being "doubled" sun conditions like reflecting infra-red off of snow or water (and in the case of water, UV, the supposed culprit, enters it and mostly does not reflect, hence the sunburned skin while snorkeling under water).

One of my other gurus, Phil Callahan, wrote the 4-page introduction to Ott's 1981 book <u>Light Radiation and You – How to Stay Healthy</u> (back when he and we did just about know about AIDS). Like Terence McKenna, Phil would agree with John Nash Ott's assertions that "Serendipidy and empirical are words that should be taken more seriously and not just shrugged off as a joke. Webster's dictionary defines serendipity as "the finding of things not sought for" and empirical as "relying on experience or observations alone without proper regard for considerations of systems, science, and theory."

Like any body part, the eye yearns for health. As I discovered in pursuing this philosophic approach also when later dealing with my triple-differently-occluded-disk back problems, the body may only be able to find its best accommodation in re-burgeoning into its genetic physicality.

Finding your way back to a text-book body norm may not be viable, but improvement of function is most certainly possible. Considering all of John Ott's practical experiments with the tangible affects of the spectrum of lighting on temperament, health, even reproduction, as a solar architect and builder, full spectrum fluorescent lighting and lots of it especially in the kitchen, have been included in all my houses. Owner/dwellers immediately feel better in their winter kitchens. Particularly pivotal in my full-spectrum lighting conversion were Ott's widely reported and influential time-lapse studies of very dramatic changes in classroom ADHD-type activity when classrooms in Rochester NY changed to full-spectrum illumination. Only implications for humans can be drawn, however, from his correct diagnosis for chinchilla breeders that the normally-balanced sex-ratios of offspring, which changed to 95% males and threatened breeding when outdoor cages were brought inside, were caused by incandescent artificial lighting, which has a high ratio of red and infrared. Changing to daylight incandescents reversed the ratio and full-spectrum lighting is now in world-wide commercial use by chinchilla breeders to maintain the number of females at 95% in the litters. Ott showed similarly that either male or female flowers can be brought forth on pumpkins by controlling slight variations in color or wave-length of light, and that the sex ratios of (live bearing) gup-pies respond similarly – many more females with daylighting.

I know, thus, that lighting effects health, but I have no conclusions for you regarding these chinchilla, flower, and fish implications for human birth gender or gender choices conceived under full-spectrum lighting. I think Ott suspected that proper healthy lighting might somehow 'feminize' humans. I don't agree with his 1973 idea that "there may be a clue here for future investigation with regard to the problem of homosexuality and the increasing number of transsexual operations." He did, however, also find and confirm that smoke-detectors and polyester bedclothes have "resulted in the loss of interest in sex today."

"If a particular ailment can be treated with certain wavelengths of light, we might logically assume that living under an artificial light source that lacks these wavelengths can contribute to causing the ailment in

the first place." "Wavelengths missing in various types of artificial light or that are filtered from the spectrum of natural light by window glass, windshields, eyeglasses (particularly tinted contact lenses or deeper shades of sunglasses), smog, and even suntan lotions, are causing a condition of malillumination, similar to malnutrition that occurs when there is a lack of a proper nutritional diet."

Lighting in the home or workplace should be re-lamped to full spectrum and, at least, compact fluorescent bulbs wherever possible (for major electrical energy savings). Full Spectrum compact fluorescent 30 Watt bulbs with a color temperature of 5500 Kelvin degrees and a Color Rendition Index (CRI) of 93 are available to provide natural outdoor lighting with an output of 2100 lumens, replacing 120 to 150 Watt bulbs and offering a life of 10,000 hours. While these may cost as much as $20 each, compared to a $3 150 Watt Sylvania soft white incandescent with 2640 lumens that lasts only 750 hours, you'ld need 13 Sylvanias at $36 total to match the compact fluorescent's 10,000 hours' longevity. $6 Full Spectrum 4 ft fluorescents - say about 4 massed and unfiltered in your kitchen ceiling as I have used them in all my houses, can also provide 9,000 lumens at 5000 Kelvin CRI 90, though the output will decline somewhat over their 20,000 hours of life. This illumination is probably enough to offset Seasonal Adsjustment Disorder with a bit of time in the kitchen.

JUST WHEN YOU THINK YOU'VE HEARD IT ALL, URINE FOR A SURPRISE

was the heading for Dr David G Williams' August 1994 Alternatives Newsmagazine sent to me by a robust man I had met at a Men's gathering who had been for 10 years part of a Water of Life group of Immune System-threatened HIV survivors in New York City. Ghandi practiced this form of Ayurvedic medicine daily. The first text my wife Alia and housemate Alilah and I read, over 20 years ago, was by a Prime Minister of India, Morarji Desai. Subsequent to our 'initiation', a woman who had been cured of a number of severe terminally ill type problems that western medicine had completely given up on gathered together the extensive research which had already been done in this country on urine therapy earlier and prior to the AMA's domination of the healing monopoly. She had found over 70 published researched scientific reports. Martha Christy used urine homeopathically and described and referenced it in her book Your Own Perfect Medicine. Indeed, **your sterile urine contains hundreds of substances that are a perfect mirror of your specific physical immune system's daily workings.** Sixty times a day your blood is edited by the kidney's computer-like library of regulatory information. The controlling software is your circadian clock. The editing program is the body's organic memory of how its genetic wholistic programming has been doing under the challenges you have been putting it to. Everything the kidney rejects is an accepted or newly to be accepted blood component, including the regulation of water.

The substances normally in your own urine have wide application for healing your epithelial tissue in a number of aspects. Skin diseases are epithelial, but so is the digestive track. Eyes are epithelial tissue and are one of the most successful areas of urine treatment, easily excelling Western medicine for eye problems like glaucoma. In WWI urine was universally recommended for sterilizing and healing open wounds. It has bacteriocidal properties. Washing your hands of your own urine is a big mistake – as well as a support of the chemical hand-emolument industry. You can apply some urine to one hand and compare the feel of the skin on each of the hands ten minutes later to discover why a major component of most skin creams is (synthetic) uric acid. But the aspect of this marvelous substance that interests me the most is its connection to viral infection. The kidney seeks to balance the pH of the blood, to regulate the balance of minerals (they rise and fall in relation to each other, you know -- you really can't build up your calcium without building up other minerals, nor will one drop severely without dragging others down), enzymes and hormones. It's all about the relationship between things. The kidneys control and retain the effective antibodies of all the viral infections that you have been exposed to and have prevailed against, like last year's flu, as well as the one you had in 1985. The kidneys have in no way forgotten 1985's challenges. And when you are exposed to this year's retro-virus (they change their form) and you begin to fight that virus and create new anti-bodies, your kidney says "not in my library -- out with it!" This is the crucial **aspect to be utilized to your advantag***e*,* through ingesting some of that sterile editing product, thus promoting the retention of vital antibodies.

For almost three decades, I have had no flu or colds. Just if the back of my throat (the "first beachhead of the virus") is inflamed in my morning inspection, as suggested by a 'scratchy' feeling on arising, the ingesting of a quarter-glass of edited kidney output stops the virus. I don't know how, exactly, and neither do the texts. But returning the antibodies back to the blood via the digestive system, or sublingually with drops under the tongue as Martha Christy recommends, just seems to do it. Traditionally the "middle morning urine" is used (salts supposedly settle to the bottom of the bladder at night and are voided first).

Our reactions to urine are pretty totally shaped by toilet training and false fastidiousness. For example, washing your hands after urinating is a big waste of hand softening because it is not really a waste product, more aptly a surplus of unneeded blood nutrients, **and your own urine is totally sterile and benign to you**. I might be misunderstood if my activism brought me to aggressively suggesting to men in toilets that they skip washing their hands, for their own good. Our disgust for urine is the result of prejudice and is conditioned by cultural influences. Its taste is not so very unpalatable. We are routinely given medicines with bitter, sharp, strange, or nauseating tastes; alcoholic drinks are often hardly pleasant to taste. In comparison, urine has a very mild and varied taste; within a few days, the artificially cultivated sense of disgust can be set aside and drinking this salty lemonade is easy. Or you could get a bunch of flue shots and, if that fails, maybe an occasional penicillin cocktail would be effective. Of course, then you'll probably still have to wait 4 days for your body to start fighting with the drug's dubious but 'statistical' help - whatever new unpredictable thing you have been exposed to. The reading for the day is from the bible: "Drink waters out of thine own cistern".

NEGATIVE ION GENERATION

Use a negative ion generator (air ionizer) to improve the quality of air in your home. Keep the generator away from computer equipment. Negative ions improve your mood and such generators create EM noise which interferes slightly with monitoring devices. Negative ions and the EM noise also counter-act negative astral and ethereal phenomena.

PHARMACEUTICAL DRUGS

Pharmaceutical drugs are another anti-nutrient category. Short term affects are usually not especially severe (if diet restores depletion), but the **nutritional affects of months or years must be taken into account**. Antibiotics, aspirin, cortisone, phenobarbitol, and tetracycline all suppress vitamin C, B vitamins, and folic acid - seen to be essential in protection from electromagnetic radiation. Here's the list:

Drug	Clinical Condition	Nutrient Affected
Antibiotics	bacterial infection	VitK, A. B12, C, K+,Mg,folicacid
Aspirin	pain, fever	VitB1, C, K+
Cortisone	inflammation,allergy	VitK+. B6, C, D, Ca, Zn, folate
Ritalin	hyperactivity, ADD	suppresses appetite
Phenobarbital	seizure disorders	Vit C, D, Ca, Mg, folic acid
Tetracycline	infection	Vit C, K, B2, B3, Zn, Ca, Fe, Mg, folate

COLLOIDAL SILVER

Colloidal silver has been used since ancient times to fight infection and eliminate disease conditions. It possesses unique germicidal properties that can interfere with the mechanisms of all bacteria, fungi, and molds, while antibiotics can typically only affect 5 or 6 species. It is a natural non-prescription antibiotic that disease systems can never develop a resistance to. The evidence is overwhelming that in the near future outbreaks of highly virulent bio-engineered diseases will occur in the populated areas of America which few people will possess the natural immunity to resist. Though the FDA tried hard to suppress it, colloidal silver can still be purchased in health food stores. Many people purchase a $110 Deluxe Colloidal Silver Generator to make all the colloidal silver you want for the cost of distilled water.

VACCINES AND EMERGING DISEASES

The dangers of vaccinations far outweigh any of their purported 'benefits'. Many victims of childhood vaccinations have resulted in death (especially SIDS) or lifelong neurological damage such as autism. Deceits, lies' and propaganda surround the promotion of vaccines. There is strong and compelling evidence that the majority of the new diseases like Ebola, Hanta Virus, Gulf War Disease, Mad Cow Disease, Red Tide, Flesh-eating Bacteria, Listeria, e-Coli, HO197, Hong Kong Bird Flu of '98, Viral Encepha-litis in Malaysia, the outbreak of the West Nile Virus in New York, the death of 25,000 Russians of TB last year, and the current "worldwide flu epidemic" have been intentionally bio-engineered by the New World Order elites for purposes of population reduction

BREAKING THE TRANCE

"Experiments conducted by researcher Herbert Krugman reveal that, when a person watches television, brain activity switches from the left to the right hemisphere. The left hemisphere is the seat of logical thought. Here, information is broken down into its component parts and critically analyzed. The right brain, however, treats incoming data uncritically, processing information in wholes, leading to emotional, rather than logical, responses. The shift from left to right brain activity also causes the release of endorphins, the body's own natural opiates - thus it is possible to become physical-ly addicted to watching television, a hypothesis borne out by numerous studies which have shown that very few people are able to kick the television habit." [Peter Russell, "Dehypnosis - Breaking the Trance"] Which does not even address the mind-fucking intent inherent to the media, in ways discernible and invisible.

THE AWARENESS ANTIDOTE

Be in the moment and observe yourself. Question baseless thoughts or emotions you may have, especially negative emotions such as aggression or depression that urge you to act without thinking. Becoming aware of their presence is often enough to deactivate them. Don't let means become ends. Reducing mind programming signal influences should serve to increase your productivity and efficiency in what you truly desire to do, the goals you chose to follow. Don't let fear and paranoia usurp the importance of following your goals.

No escape - Geomagnetic Energy Changed by

60 Hz Power Lines and Background Radiation

Aurora are a manifestation of Gaia's magnetism. Earth is wrapped in a magnetic field -- a donut-shaped enclosure that extends hundreds of miles out into space; Earth itself is at the donut's hole. **Geomagnetism** envelopes Earth with circular lines of flux which descend at the North Pole, penetrate through Earth's center to emerge at the South Pole, then loop out through space in vast circles that return to the North.

Geomagnetism wraps the earth in a protective magnetic shield to deflect dangerous radiation away from fragile life-forms in Gaia's biosphere. Solar winds of high energy particles sweep at our planet and are diverted by the geomagnetic field. Gaia's magnetic cloak also **shapes the ionsphere**, a thin upper air layer ionized by ultraviolet radiation to form the now well-known ozone layer. On the sun side, solar winds compress the magnetosphere to about 10 earth radii and increase its magnitude. On the dark side, solar winds expand the magnetosphere so it billows into a wind-sock like structure called the magnetotail, which stretches over 1,000 earth radii. **The magnetosphere looks like a dragon**, with compact head facing the sun and a very long tail streaming out into stellar darkness (and opening us much more to cosmic energy).

Periodically, the Sun erupts with flares -- gigantic tongues of flaming plasma which shoot thousands of miles into space. These solar plumes emit bursts of charged particles to create **shockwaves** in the solar wind which bombards our planet. The geomagnetic turbulence this generates interferes significantly with radio and satellite communications, as well as with powerlines and defense systems.

During solar storms, gusts of charged particles captured in geomagnetism spiral along flux lines to ice capped poles. Only 20 years ago science found that as captive electron beams stream through polar air, they collide with gas molecules to ionize atoms, causing them to glow in momentary energy release. The invisible becomes visible -- Gaia's magnetic cloak is revealed in its luminous glory as solar storms stream energy pulses through Earth's polar vortexes.

Gaia's twin auroral wreaths are thus children of heaven and earth. Both the Earth's magnetic mantle and the Sun's bursts of electric particles are needed to ignite auroral displays. This does not, however, explain them.

One of the prophets of free energy, Nikola Tesla, is revered for his invention of **radiant energy technology** whereby electricity can be converted to remote locations without the use of wires. His work was usurped by HAARP and he died a man broken by the hegemony, unable to prevent the deadly purposes to which it had applied his creative energies [*see Appendixes in All-That-Is Waving on Montauk and the Philadelphia Experiments of the early 1940s.*]. HAARP has sufficient strength signals to turn the aurora borealis into a virtual antenna, re-broadcasting in the ELF range, which can travel deep into the earth, as well as through us - with very immanent dangers.

On the Earth's surface, America is crisscrossed today by spiderwebs of radiant energy, emitted while supplying electricity to millions of factories and homes with dozens of lights, motors, appliances, and gadgets. At night billions of street lights, stop lights and neon ads drive back the dark. [I saw <u>Koyanisquatski</u> again recently. Its time-lapse photography of the electrical/light web of great cities at night is a dramatic depiction of this rampant energy.] **There is no place in the U S that does not have background radiation frequencies from high-power lines. Radio, telephones, TV, and computers revolutionized science, business and communications. Microwaves cook fast food and beam wideband data channels to distant sites via orbiting satellite. Radar tracks movement on earth or in air, including cars with cellular phones and CB radios.**

Radiation exposure

Most of the radiation the general public is exposed to comes from natural sources, such as cosmic rays and radioactive elements in the Earth's crust.

Sources of radiation exposure in U.S.

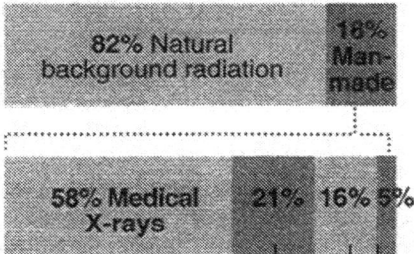

82% Natural background radiation | 18% Man-made

58% Medical X-rays | 21% | 16% | 5%

Nuclear medicine – Use of radioactive isotopes in diagnosis or treatment

Consumer products (tobacco, domestic water supply, building materials, etc.)

Occupational exposure, fallout, nuclear fuel cycle

SOURCES: National Academy of Sciences; EPA   AP

The National Academy of Sciences panel (8/05) rejected the extended nuclear industry claim of low radiation levels being not harmful, possibly even beneficial. It stated 3.1/millisevert (measure of radiation energy) per year is deposited in living tissue from background radiation, when 100 millisevert of radiation over a lifetime introduces the odds of solid cancer or leukemia, with half those cases being final.

A whole body CAT scan introduces 10 millisevert. **At 3.1/yr background radiation alone, without including microwaves from appliances, cell phones, high tension wires in the mix, a little dose of 32 years'll do ya for fifty-fifty chances. "There is no threshold below which radiation can be viewed as harmless". Eighteen percent of the ambient radiation of the planet is created by our unthinking and irresponsible species.**

Today, 600,000 miles of power lines crisscross the U.S., with thousands more planned or in construction. This entire power grid is a giant ELF antenna whose pulsating magnetic field spans the continent. How this man-made EM affects other organisms and larger ecosystems - or earth as a whole - is sorely understudied and poorly understood. Yet its affect is easily discernable in the news, which never examines the implications of what it reports.

What makes trees grow up is magnetism. A tree is a dipole antenna to focus and harness geomagnetism in soil and rock. Plants materialize this spinning vortex of magnetism. Magnetism affects water in odd ways. Normally water's pH is neutral due to its balance of acid (H+) to alkaline (OH-) ions. But south pole magnetism causes water to become slightly alkaline, while north pole shifts pH slightly acid. This subtle shift is critical in biological systems such as cell membranes. Cells must resonate a full range of geomantic frequencies for mitosis and meiosis to occur. **The DNA is a super-coiled antenna tuned to high frequency short wave oscillations. Iron red in hemoglobin and cobalt blue in vitamin B12 are a magnetic wave form chalice to transport electrons in blood and nerve. Like quartz in Gaia's granite mantle, human bone is a piezoelectric crystal oscillating at precise resonant frequencies.**

RESEARCH HISTORY

In 1982 Robert Becker and Andrew Marino, leading medical researchers in bioelectromagnetics, published <u>Electromagnetism and Life</u>, whose Preface stated: "But the coin has another side. The environment is now thoroughly polluted by man-made EM with frequencies and magnitudes never before present. Man's activities probably changed earth's EM background to a greater degree than any other natural attribute -- whether land, water or atmosphere. Evidence indicates abnormal EM environments constitute a health risk. Today interest in all facets of this is at an unprecedented pitch." **The power grid is actually damaging the earth by disrupting the natural flow of its aetheric geomagnetic energy.**

In 1974, Dr. Nancy Wertheimer began a significant study in Denver that linked power-line magnetism to childhood leukemia. Now, after two decades, a vast body of research has revealed **man-made electromagnetism (EM) adversely affects** many delicate biological processes: **bone growth, cell communication, biocycles, blood cells, neurochemistry, genetic replication,**

immune system, and more. Today the weight of evidence reveals our consumption EM genie is assaulting us on all fronts.

In Jan. 1980 Dr. Ross Adey of UCLA's Brain Research Institute spoke on biological effects of microwaves at the Amer. Assoc. for the Advancement of Science's annual meeting. Studies showed magnetism pulsed at 15 or 72 Hz **altered parathyroid hormone action** to trigger adenylate cyclase, a cell membrane enzyme **<u>crucial to forming new bone</u>**. External EM is too weak to alter cell chemistry, so cell membranes must sense weak EM to trigger changes in cell behavior. Adey pointed out this EM is similar to radar, and blasted the Air Force for failure to honestly assess its EM emission risks.

By 1982 Adey showed how 450 MHz radar modulated at 60 Hz greatly reduced T-lymphocyte activity to kill cultured cancer cells. Adey's associate Daniel Lyle replicated the study using powerline 60 Hz, and found major declines in T-lymphocyte activity. A 1983 report noted smaller effects occur at 40, 16 and three Hz where the brain operates in resonance with Schumann waves. This **had serious implications for millions of people living near powerlines**.

Under pressure, Air Force gave $4 million to study long-term effects of low-level microwaves. Profs. Guy and Chou, engineers at Univ. of Washington Bioelectromagnetics Lab, exposed 100 rats to continuous low level microwaves for two years to examine effects on blood chemistry, body weight and behavior. Results released in Aug. 1984 were shocking: 16 malignant tumors in exposed rats versus only four in controls; seven in exposed rats were endocrine, one in controls.

In 1983 Craig Byrus, biomedicine professor at U. of California at Riverside, exposed human tonsil lymphcytes to low level 450 MHz modulated at ELF from three to 100 hz for up to 60 minutes. He found protein-kinase enzymes became inacive at specific frequencies between 16 and 60 hz; protein-kinase C is a receptor for cancer-promoting substances. Printed in 1984 in Bioelectromagnetics, this raised disturbing questions about effects of ELF and microwaves on the human immune system, our first line of defense against cancer. **Our national defense's EM sensing technology was now implicated in damage to our personal biological defenses**.

THIS WAS FOLLOWED BY A DECADE OF DENIAL

Clearly something was happening. Here was repeated, credible evidence of public health hazards associated with EM exposure, but the effect had an unknown cause. Fingers of evidence in this mystery pointed at magnetism, but no one could explain how low-level magnetism causes cell disorder or disease.

Hector D Perez Torres of Advanced Research Knowledge asserts that "Power company lines act as a sink for naturally occurring Radio Frequency RF energy waves in low to very low frequencies (LF/VLF) from 19 KHz to 535 KHz/". Because of known interactions between naturally occurring earth VLF frequencies emitted from the earth, "they invert lines at intervals and place filters and suppressors in line" to counter these effects. "Utility companies expend millions in filtering geodesic 'noise' that affects their system, like in solar storms."

AFFECTS OF MAGNETIC FIELDS

Perhaps the most dangerous, damaging form of pollution facing Americans every minute of every day is invisible, soundless, and cannot be touched or felt (well, I get a headache after standing 5 minutes under the high voltage wires at the foot of Long Hill Rd near my house. And I don't get headaches.). It is electromagnetic field radiation (EMF) and it is emanating from virtually every single electrical appliance, computer, electric wire, and especially high voltage lines - both overhead and buried - which are carrying current. EMF is specifically causing cancer in children and older adults and may be triggering countless other immune deficiency and psychological diseases and disorders in anyone in close proximity. Make no mistake about it: electrical fields are bad news for health and can be killers.

A massive study by the Swedish government of the effects of electrical fields from overhead power lines on 500,000 people over a period of 25 years found overwhelming evidence that electric fields generated cancer in children at 4 times the normal rate and tripled the rate in adults. Sweden lists electromagnetic fields as Class 2 Carcinogens, right along with tobacco.

In Edgehouse, I included a picture of 1,300 8-ft fluorescent tubes stuck in the ground under 50 Hz high voltage lines. This sculpture in England by Richard Box raised my 39-year awareness of proximity to high voltage lines in sight of my house to a concern for the seven families across the street from Edgehouse who for **four generations have lived in the Right Of Way of a pair of high-voltage lines and manifest many alarming, especially when considered in the aggregate, physical ailments.** I purchased a Tri-Field Meter, which measures microwaves [which 'cook'] and Radio frequencies, magnetic fields [measured in milligauss], and electrical fields [measured in kilovolts per meter]. The readings near and under the power lines were more than alarming, with 17 kilovolts per meter - or 17,000 volts per meter under one of the lines and 1,500 volts per meter or greater where the houses are located.

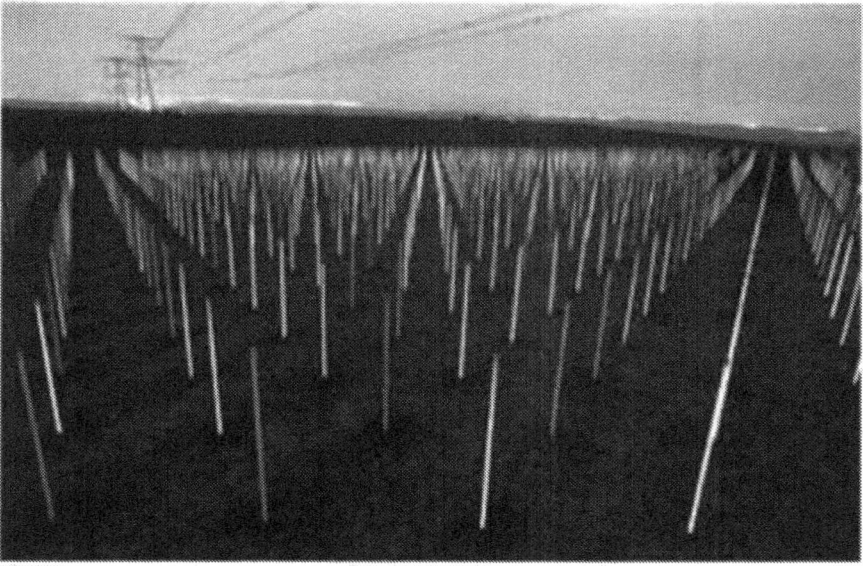

To simply demonstrate this concern, I executed an inverted tetrahedron of 8-ft fluorescent tubes under the line. I chose the inverted tetrahedron form which, you will remember, is the form of the platonic solid that is the basic building block of manifestation - in largest energy form with its point in the center of the earth providing the triangular patterns of energy and tension to the earth's crust.

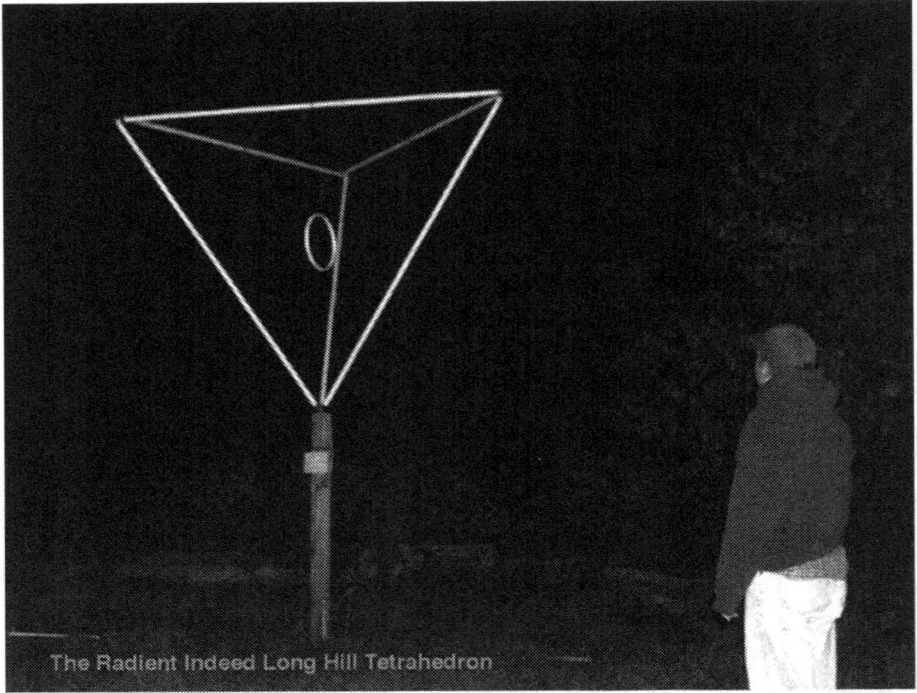

The Radient Indeed Long Hill Tetrahedron

Many scientists warn people not to live within 200 yards of high voltage power lines. Of 35 international research studies on electric field radiation, 33 established a conclusive link between brain tumors, leukemia, and other forms of cancer. Other studies report clear linkage between EMF exposure and illnesses such as immune disorders, brain wave modification, and many other serious physical and psychological abnormalities and deficiencies.

Russian scientists have been studying EMF more than any other country and have been reporting that electrical fields cause high blood pressure, changes in white and red blood cell counts, increased metabolism, chronic fatigue disorders, and headaches.

There are 20 - 70 million chronic insomniacs in the US and millions more who sleep poorly. Many researcher and scientists now feel that **electromagnetic field radiation, both from within and without the bedroom, is the single biggest factor in poor sleep.** And poor health. Look around the bedroom.

Is there a clock radio on the nightstand near your pillow? A TV? A stereo? Do you see an electric blanket**? Are there high voltage lines near your residence?** All or any of these electric sources can ruin your sleep and can substantially increase your risk of developing cancer and any number of diseases, both psychological and physical. While you sleep, your body relaxes and is unconscious. In this state of vulnerability, research indicates you are 100-150 times more open to the damage of electromagnetic radiation than when you are awake. It can take hours for the built up voltage in even an unplugged TV to dissipate. A clock near your head can cause health problems. Electric blankets (nobody uses them any more because of the dangers, do they?) radiate fields over 70,000 times higher than normal acceptable levels.

In 1976, Dr. Ross Adey of UCLA's Brain Research Institute proved that weak EM directly affects the central nervous system, and theorized that ELF oscillations of protein-calcium strands are cell-to-cell communication. **Weak ELF EM alters calcium movement in cell membranes including the brain and bones to change neural chemical action.**

The pineal gland is now believed to be the master endocrine gland, yielding a pharmacopoia of psychoactive chemicals to regulate all our glands. It also secretes neurohormones - *melatonin, serotonin, dopamine* - to regulate brain operations. The sleep-wake cycle depends on the level of pineal *melatonin.* *Melatonin* **secretion can be changed by magnetic exposure at the level of geomagnetism. The pineal is our magnetic gland to read geomagnetic pulsations and translate them to hormones to drive our biocycles.** This suggests how ELF can disrupt our biorhythms.

From the power company I learned that the western power row of the 2 across the road from me is not in service. It is a back-up to the substation that is only activated by emergency need. **The Eastern line is a 115kV** supposedly rated according to the Manual at 29,700 vpm under it [The power company guy got 28,000 vpm at the top of the hill], and 6,500 vpm 50 ft away and 1,700 vpm 100 ft away. When we took measurements, his meter consistently recorded higher than what my Tri-field meter did. My lower measurements of the not-functioning western row it turns out were simply of distances from the influence of the active adjacent 115 kV eastern line. The large center line grounded to the towers is a fiber optic line. The top wire is a grounding wire between towers, which is matched by an underground wire between the towers. On each side, the arms hold three lines of different polarity making two 'circuits'. [That must mean two hot lines and a neutral, which takes power when it needs to balance the two live loads.]

I have been measuring electromagnetic radiation with my Tri-field meter, which is a combine of electrical and magnetic radiation. "Electric loads are relatively stable from power lines, but magnetic fields fluctuate as current changes in response to changing loads." When I switched the meter dial from 'electric' to 'magnetic' the readings were the same.

From the Manuel I skipped here: "The International Commission on Non-Ionizing Radiation Protection sets guidelines for EMF Exposure for occupational at 8,000 vpm electric and 4,200 milligauss magnetic. For the General Public it states 4,200 vpm electric and 833 milligauss. The American Conference of Governmental Industrial Hygienists states that workers with **cardiac pacemakers should not be exposed to 60 Hz magnetic field greater than 1,000 milligauss or a 60 Hz electrical field greater than 1,000 vpm**."

A man living at the end of the row of 7 houses 1500 ft away from me in a house I measured outside at 1,500 vpm, has had a quadruple bypass and had to replace four pacemakers. Also a replaced knee, I believe. His 40-something son who grew up with my children had a stroke and is half paralyzed and has difficulty recognizing his parents. A son at the other end of the row of houses who went to school with my kids died from unknown (to me) causes in his forties. Late 2006 his mother died. In January 2007 his same-aged cousin died of cancer. Six of the seven families are related and genetics (over 4 generations under the lines) may be primary in at least 7 hip replacements in 3 men of the 2 older generations. Calcium in bones and brain transfer are, however, clearly proven to be affected by electromagnetic radiation. The second and third generations of both genders are all very heavy and 5 of the generation that went to school with my family seem somewhat handicapped.

All of this is what I have observed and I know nothing of the incidence of cancer or other medical problems of this extended family that has lived in over 1000 vpm since 1924. I'm pretty sure, however, that almost everyone there has had a lot of contact with the medical establishment. Was radiation considered by the doctors?

I have asked my neighbors' forgiveness for invading their privacy. Even though the original family homestead was somehow brought from a mountain 8 miles away in 1795 and the other 6 residences all have been built since I have lived here in 1966, I know they are not going to move. Having aggressively taken my health into my own hands about 5 years ago and wrested any control or involvement other than physicals away from the Four Horsemen of the Apothecary, the only thing I could do to enhance their relationship with a life in perpetual radiation was to research what I could find and suggest **an appropriate nutritional supplementation that could lead to restoring hormonal balance and bolstering the immune system to counteract the continual Electromagnetic stress. This was hard to find.**

Food Prana Supplementation

It had been made clear in a number of studies that **EMF/RF Radiation mandates B12 and Folic Acid supplementation.** I have come to assume that everybody knows about this one, which medicine also recommends for homocystiene/cholesterol reduction. My doctor recommended these, along with Vitamin B6 after my angina attacks 9 years ago. [In a recent Harvard study, women with the highest blood levels of Vitamin B-6 had a 58 and 44 percent reduced risk of colon and colorectal cancer respectively, compared to those with the lowest levels.**] Folate deficiency** has been talked about since Michio Kushi had broccoli from the supermarkets tested for it in the 80s and found B-12 and Folic Acid levels depleted from green and yellow veggies by american agriculture. Macrobiotics guru Michio Kushi recommended natural sources for Vitamin C, B vitamins and Folate for cancer, and the avoidance of all fatty animal foods, oils, and greases.[I particularly remember in connection with this that broccoli was the one food that George the First wouldn't eat.] Folate deficiency may correlate with development of alcoholic polyneuropathy (it's a liver detox). University of California researchers have found that 400 mcg of folic acid cuts the risk of Alzheimers in half. I take 1.2 mg/day. Life Extension Foundation recommends from 800 to 5,000 mcg (.8 - 5 mg)/ day. **[LEF recommendations below are for everyone daily, not those indicated for cancer treatment]**

Humans and all vertebrates require *cobalt*, though it is assimilated only in the form of Vitamin B12 - *cyancobalanin*

B-12 is for heart, energy metabolism and immune and nerve function, mental functioning and mood. B12, in the form of *methylcobalamin*, taken in lozenge form dose of 5 to 40 mg/day sublingually, along with 2 to 5 mg of folic acid has been shown to correct many neurological diseases including neuropathy. B12 is the only vitamin synthesized solely by certain microorganisms - many of which are abundant in soil. And the only vitamin containing a trace element: *cobalt*. B12 owes its chemical name - *cobalamin* - to *cobalt* at the center of its molecular structure,. I take 1,125 mcg daily.

Cobalt is **one of the three naturally magnetic elements** (the others are Iron, essential to biological systems, and Nickel - toxic to most organisms). ***Cobalt's*** magnetic geometry plays a crucial role in electron transfers, allowing a cell to spin an electron and transform its electric charge to magnetic flux. In animal tissue, B-12 concentrates in the kidneys, liver, and heart, but its highest concentration is **in the pineal gland, where this cobalt-rich radio-transmitter is our central sensor of seasonal change and controls our circadian rhythms.**

Bacteria on the root nodules of legumes require *cobalt* to synthesize B-12 and fix nitrogen from the air. But soil bacteria - 20% of soil biomass - are destroyed or inactivated by ag chemicals, inhibiting uptake and metabolism of *cobalt* and other **trace elements of the glacial legacy, which are in precipitous decline.** Vegetarians absolutely must supplement this essential vitamin. It is relatively little known that the Tobacco grown by native Americans was an essential B vitamin food source, used in soups to supplement corn, beans, and squash which have no B-12. The Four Horsemen of the Apothecary had to separate this B vitamin out from the B's hive because it was the only one of the B vitamins they couldn't synthesize from petroleum and profit from.

The only source I could find for natural diet supplementation to combat the affect of living in an electromagnetic field even more extreme than the surrounding 60 cycle network grid that is in fact omnipresent in each residence was the <u>Adjuvant Cancer</u> recommendations of the **Life Extension Foundation** - the largest non-profit research organization in the world focussed on the area between conventional medicine and natural nutrition and supplementation. Their only Protocol Reference regarding the dangers of radiation was on ameliorating the affect of radiation therapy. I found a number of supplements on their list of anti-oxidants to help prevent cancer cells from developing resistance to radiation therapy that are already on my carefully crafted regime for health, and several with which I am unfamiliar.

Vitamin E - gamma E tocopherols protect against free-radical damage, coronary disease, immune system, leg cramps. [Now coupled with 1,000 mg life-extending **L-Carnosine**, for long-lived neurons and muscle cells, heart-efficient enhanced calcium response, skin elasticity, vision] I take 466 IU. LEF recommended 2 x 400 IU/day

Melatonin LEF suggests 20 mg nightly. I also use a tryptamine serotonin precurser **5 HTP**, potentiated by 500 mg of **L-Tyrosine**, a precursor to norepinephrine. **5 HTP** has also been **an antidepressant for decades in Europe that outperforms Prozac** w/ dosage of 100 mg 3x/day. I take 200 mg before sleep to improve REM and perhaps lucid dreaming.

Vitamin C - Antioxidant protection, inhibits the oxidation of LDL cholesterol build-up. I take 1,000 mg time-release with rose hips that cover 8 hours twice a day. LEF recommended 4 to 12 g/day in divided doses (Vitamin C normally leaves the blood in several hours and is therefore given intravenously in hospitals.) Whenever the back of the throat signals a new infection, increasing the dosage of these time-release Cs (along with a touch of Urine Therapy, which has kept me totally free of colds or flus for 30 years) will stop the infection.

Taurine - A derivative of cysteine, an amino acid, Taurine protects against free radicals between cells, eye lens against oxidation, vision. LEF recommended 2,000 mg daily. I take 500 mg at night <u>on an empty stomach</u>. It works together with **Acetyl L-**

Carnitine on muscle weakness, general fatigue, cramps, aches, during renal dialysis - renal problems - retinopathy. In conjunction with Taurine, **CoQ10 enzyme**, **magnesium**, **chromium**, and **potassium** may be beneficial to congestive heart failure. High intakes of fish oil improves function. I take 2 x 500 mg L-Carnitine /day.

The amino acid cysteine is inherent in the 2 drugs/supplements that LEF suggested **to reduce the side affects and damages caused by radiation** therapy:

Se-methylselenocysteine (SeMSC), was suggested at 200-400 mcg/day and **N-Acetyl-cysteine (NAC)** at 600 mg 1x/day. They also suggested **Whey Protein concentrate isolate** 10 - 20 grams 3x/day.

I think **L-Arginine**, a nitric oxide synthase enzyme involved in vascular homeostasis, immune regulation, and host defense and blood carrying capacities should definitely be included by everyone. It nourishes muscle tissue to enhance strength and endurance. LEF recommends 500-1,000 mg daily with water, taken at night. I take 500 mg before bed.

If this stimulates an examination of your supplementation, I would also most vehemently recommend everyone's balancing of their **DHEA** , with a natural substance (made from a wild Mexican yam) that **supplements shortage of the most common hormone in the body,** a natural steroid which protects the heart, grows brain cells, is anti-aging, bone building, and burns fat to lose weight and convert fat to muscle. **Every older male must balance out DHEA levels in the body to youthful levels as production plummets with age so that at age 70 less than 20 percent of this essential testosterone precursor is produced by the male body! It regulates weight**. Three years ago I lost 25 lbs in a month and regained lost vital energy. I attribute this primarily to this testosterone precursor's balancing in older age. The regulation of my weight continues in place even when I 'overeat' for days. Females may not need any DHEA supplementation, but LEF's newly discovered component of **DHEA 7-Keto** is a proven weight controller that does not change testosterone levels in women.

Pursuing this weight control aspect further, I consulted on line ConsumerHealthDigest.com's review of the top 30 weight loss products for metabolism enhancement, weight loss potential, appetite suppression, and ingredient quality. The top nine were rated from 96 points out of 100 down to 91/100, with weight loss 5 of 5 down to 4 of 5. The top product, Lipovarin, with *a proprietary formula,* "targets fat loss from many different angles" and includes the **7-Keto** component of **DHEA**, isolated by LEF 2 years ago, described as "stimulating the enzymes in the liver responsible for thermogenesis, increasing the body's metabolic efficiency, greater weight loss results, and **maintaining ideal body weight**." **Caffeine** and **Green Tea** are included to "stimulate thermogenic and metabolic effects as well as **supporting increases in resting energy expenditure." Theobromine** - Cacao chocolate - "provides a thermogenic effect and euphoric feeling." **Citrus auranticum**, also **called Neroli/Bitter Orange** blossom flower oil, is "similar to Ma Huang, without negative side effects", suppressing hunger. **Coral Calcium, Taurine, and Gloconolactone** support the functionality of other key ingredients. Along with **Serotain** "for appetite suppression" - an extract of *Griffonia simplifolia* and source for **5-H T P** which boosts *Serotonin* levels, as listed earlier. The above ingredients make up this very successful *proprietary formula*, called "Metazide". They are basically most of what was suggested earlier.

For health, you also should also investigate **Essential Fatty Acids - the Omega oils** that are missing from our diets. They improve the health of the arteries, curb inflammation and plaque growth.

And, of course, a carefully derived Multi Vitamin like local Pioneer Nutritional Formulas' **VITAMIN MINERAL SUPPLEMENT** available at Whole Foods or Green Field's Market, should be included by everyone to provide dozens of essential trace minerals missing from foods, along with other vitamin and nutrient supplementation. This too, is important.

A slight caution on vitamin mineral supplementation, however appropriate the initial titration dosages may have been. You need to stay aware of the supplemental details including the multi- in your ongoing protocol of adjuvenation. My one or the other or in tandem inner calf muscles' nightly crampdown, usually eventually released by going 'on point', as it were, was discredited to have been gout or enthusiastic wine drinking or the result of neuropathy and lastly checked in for being too B-Sixed! Stopping the 500 mg in Balanced-B supplement didn't fix it, but the day I stopped the multiple vitamin I had initially built my repair schedule around, with it's 450 mg of B-6, the crampout fires were doused.

CONTENTS

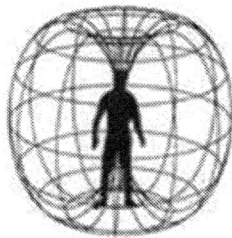

www.ingramcontent.com/pod-product-compliance
Lightning Source LLC
Chambersburg PA
CBHW031519270326
41930CB00006B/432